ANGLES OF REFLECTION

LOGIC AND

A MOTHER'S LOVE

Joan L. Richards

W. H. FREEMAN AND COMPANY · NEW YORK

Text design: Diana Blume

Library of Congress Cataloging-in-Publication Data

Richards, Joan L., 1948–
    Angles of reflection: logic and a mother's love/Joan L. Richards.
    p. cm.
    ISBN 0-7167-3831-7
    1. Richards, Joan L., 1948– 2. Mothers—Rhode Island—Providence—
Biography. 3. College teachers—Rhode Island—Providence—Biography.
4. Mathematics historians—Rhode Island—Providence—Biography.
5. Sabbatical leave—Germany—Case studies. 6. Tumors in children—
Case studies. 7. Brain—Tumors—Case studies. I. Title.
HQ759.R535 2000
306.874'3'092—dc21
[B]
                                                                00-024875

Printed in the United States of America

First printing 2000

W. H. Freeman and Company
41 Madison Avenue, New York, NY 10010
Houndmills, Basingstoke RG21 6XS, England

For my mother, Victoria H. Campbell,
who has always led the way.

Contents

Part I
Fuzzy Vision, Enhanced Vision

Grand Mal

I don't remember when I got the letter inviting me to spend a year at the *Wissenschaftskolleg* in Berlin. There certainly was no question that I would accept it. I had for the previous seven years poured myself into my family. My husband was engulfed with work at the Rhode Island Department of Education, I by the day-by-day demands of my job as a professor of the history of science at Brown University. The combination of raising two children and working in an institution that took undergraduate teaching seriously meant that I had long neglected "my work," my research and writing.

Not engaging it had its own set of negative consequences, however. Somehow I had managed to teach and finish my dissertation after Brady, my first child, was born. I finished my first book when Ned, my second child, was still in diapers. But my second book had not followed as expected. Raising two children had proved itself to be just too distracting to allow me to think through a whole new project. Though I scheduled a full workload around them—teaching, serving on committees, delivering papers—I could not muster the kind of total concentration required to write. Six years into my tenure, my department turned down my promotion. I could not refute their objection that I had not written a second book. What I could do was recognize that at nine and fourteen the boys were no longer as demanding as they had been before, and it was high time to concentrate on my research and writing.

So, when my sabbatical finally came due, I put all of my energies into finding ways to extend with outside money the one semester I was granted. I had been successful and had a fellowship at the Dibner Institute in Cambridge, Massachusetts. The fellowship gave me a lovely office overlooking the Charles River in the midst of a group of people whose interests overlapped with mine. Working in the institute required that I commute, itself a privilege because it placed distance between my personal and my work life. Three or four mornings a week I left the house by seven-fifteen to catch the train to Boston, returning between five and five-thirty. In between my fellowship granted me time, space, and colleagues—a whole world for my work. It was wonderful.

The *Wissenschaftskolleg* offered yet more of the same—another year and another place in which to do my work. It required considerably more in terms of dislocation—the year would be in Berlin. I had never been to Germany for more than a week, my most recent contact with the language was a course, "German for Reading Knowledge," taken for my Ph.D. exams more than twenty years before. But I knew that for my work it didn't really matter where I was. A year in Germany would be a broadening adventure for the whole family. So, I am sure that I was thrilled when I got the letter offering me the fellowship and equally sure that I wrote back to accept with alacrity. But I do not remember now. At just about the time that it arrived my family was engulfed in a series of events that has blocked the specifics of the letter and my response entirely from my mind.

The scenes I do remember from that fall begin in a dark kitchen. It was about five-thirty in the evening on November 9 when I trundled up the back stairs, back from a long day in Cambridge. No lights were on, and I missed the conversation, music, arguments, and tromping around that the family could usually be counted on to provide. Bilbo, our black cocker spaniel, came hopefully into the kitchen but all else seemed still. Then I heard footsteps from Brady's far-away room. He was in a sequestered phase, which explained why the apartment seemed so deserted even though he was there.

As he came toward me the telephone rang, and Brady intercepted it. "Yes," he said. "She just came home. Yes, I'll get her."

"It's Dad," he said as he handed it to me. "He's in the hospital with Ned."

In the hospital with Ned? It was a strange concept. Ned was exuberantly healthy—perhaps he had fallen and broken a limb. I took the phone.

Rick sounded quite normal. "Ned and I need a ride home," he said. "Can you come pick us up?"

"Sure," I said, "but where are you?"

"I'm in a neurologist's office," he replied. "Ned had some kind of seizure at school. He's fine now though, and we are ready to come home. Brady can tell you about it, and I'll explain more when you come, but Dr. Gasparian's office is closing. Can you pick us up?" he repeated.

"Yes," I said but I had no idea where a neurologist's office might be. Rick gave me instructions and Brady and I went to the car.

As we drove the unfamiliar streets to the downtown Providence hospital complex I pumped my taciturn adolescent for information. He did not know a great deal but told what he could. "Ned had some kind of a fit in the lunchroom at school. I guess they couldn't reach you in Boston but they told Dad. He came to school and went in the ambulance with Ned. I think things got kind of screwed up at the hospital, but basically everything is fine now."

"Ned had a fit?" I asked. "What do you mean a fit? Did he have a temper tantrum?"

"No, Mom. You don't go to the hospital for a temper tantrum. I don't know what kind of fit—how should I know?"

It seemed a reasonable position. I peered through the rainy night, trying to follow Rick's directions through this unfamiliar part of town, finally locating the appropriate parking lot. Brady slumped his rapidly growing self in the front seat, knees on the dashboard. "Leave the keys. I'll listen to the radio," he said.

I left him there and followed Rick's directions to the third floor of a dreary office building where I found the nondescript offices of "Dr. Gasparian, Neurology." The secretary indicated a room in the back when I asked about my husband and child.

I found Rick and Ned in a small, white room. Ned flashed me his irresistible smile from a cross-legged perch on an examining table. He looked absolutely fine except for a large bruise half-hidden under the thick, light-brown hair on his forehead. Rick was sitting in one of two chairs on the other side of the room. He looked uncharacteristically disheveled: shirt dirty, pants crumbled, tie askew. His carefully trimmed beard was wilted. His usually neat gray hair bushed Einstein-like from his forehead. The eyes behind his horn-rimmed glasses were weary. A large poster of the brain, all brown-gray scrolls and little red labels, covered the wall behind him.

"What happened, Sweetie?" I sat in the other chair.

Rick leaned his shoulder tiredly against me. "Oh, Joan, I wish I knew. The school called me out of a meeting to say that Ned had had a seizure in the lunchroom. You had the car, so I got a cab and went as fast as I could. Ned was unconscious. We went in an ambulance to the hospital. Just about when we got there Ned threw up, all over everything. There were doctors everywhere. They tried to get Dr. Johnson, but he was out of the office. So they hooked Ned up to all sorts of machines, took blood, ordered a CAT scan, decided an EEG would be better and left us in a little room. That was about three and I guess the shifts changed. We just sat and watched TV. They didn't notice us again until it was five and we had missed the EEG. They sent us to Dr. Gasparian's anyway, so here we are. But his office is closed; he's not going to do it now."

"I banged my head on the table!" Ned said brightly. "See my bruise?"

When I had been briefed to this extent, we were interrupted by a slight, dark-complexioned man. There were introductions all around and then Dr. Gasparian asked me whether I could shed further light on Ned's condition. "Your son had a convulsive seizure at about noon today. Has anything like this ever happened before?"

My first reaction was "No," but as I turned it over in my mind I realized that might be too glib. Last spring Ned had once been sent home from school because something odd had happened. When he came in from recess, he said, the room went dark and he began to walk into furniture. The teacher told him to put his head on his desk and he did, but he got such a bad headache he could not concentrate. So, she sent him to the principal's office and they called me to fetch him. When I arrived, Ned had a splitting headache. Thinking that the problem might be that he had become dehydrated at recess, I gave him a glass of water. Then I supported him for the six-block walk home. When we got there I put him to bed in a darkened room, but he was already almost completely recovered. I could not keep him down for more than half an hour; the water had worked its magic.

The second incident was less noticeable. About a month before, when I had picked him up at the end of the school day, Ned had a terrible headache—he was shrunken into his body with great circles under his eyes. He said that he had had some trouble seeing in his last class, but it was not bad enough that anyone noticed. I treated him gently and he was totally normal by dinnertime.

I had told Rick about each of these episodes when it happened, but they were so minor that he had not registered them. They had been fleeting incidents, of no more moment than any of a myriad of other childhood ups and downs. I felt almost disloyal reconstructing them as seizures while the strange doctor gravely took notes and probed Ned for corroboration or clarification.

"We'll have to do an EEG as soon as possible," Dr. Gasparian said, and made an appointment for Friday afternoon. "I also need to know as much as possible about what happened today and on these other days. Ask the teachers or Ned's classmates what they remember, anything, and bring the information with you when you come."

I wanted to know more—about convulsive seizures, about an EEG, about the whole situation. How normal was a seizure? What caused them? Who had them? Why? What was an EEG? Would it hurt Ned? What would it show? How was Ned now? Did we need to do anything special? All of these questions and more filled my head, but Dr. Gasparian was not a man to chat. He showed us firmly to the door with a card showing Ned's EEG appointment on Friday, two days away.

In Dr. Gasparian's office Rick was calm, but on the car ride home it became clear that he had been deeply shaken. Nothing in the call that jerked him from a meeting at work had prepared him to find Ned unconscious. His own child had looked at him but not responded in any way. He had not grinned or even blinked when Rick spoke to him; he had not returned the pressure when Rick took his hand. Eyes open, he had lain blank and still on the couch in the nurse's office.

Rick was overwhelmed, but hardly more so than the school personnel who had summoned him. The story they told was simply weird. It seemed that when the children were dismissed for recess, there was a disturbance at the table where Ned had been sitting. When the lunchroom supervisor went to investigate she found that several children had dreamed up a new way to misbehave by taking refuge under the complex structure that combined table and chairs. She firmly told them to come out, which they all willingly did—all but Ned who ignored her and continued to wiggle on the floor. Irritated, she reached in to pull him out. It was only when his arm jerked uncontrollably in her grasp that she realized that she was dealing with more than a creatively naughty child. She then registered Ned's eyes rolling back into his head, his mouth alternately drooling and tensing, his head rhythmically pounding against the leg of the table. Horrified, she called for assistance. By the time another teacher arrived, Ned had stopped moving, but he was so tangled in the supports of the table and chairs that they could not pull him out. More teachers arrived: some shooed the crowd of entranced classmates onto the playground while others tried to figure out what to do with the limp child under the table. Ultimately they extricated Ned by lifting up the whole table-and-chair structure, thus allowing him to fall out onto the floor. They then carried him to the nurses' office where Rick found him.

When the ambulance arrived there was something to do besides stare at the comatose Ned. The emergency medical technicians briskly transferred Ned into their vehicle and made a place for Rick to sit beside him. Rick held Ned's wrist with its comforting pulse all of the way to the hospital; it was the only indication he had that Ned was not dead. He confessed he had never been so relieved as when Ned threw up all over him.

At home we ate a simple supper. Ned was completely exhausted and went to bed, Brady retreated to his room, and Rick fled to the paper in the living room. I went to the kitchen and the dishes. "What is happening to my little boy? What is the matter with Ned?" I asked the little cherub in a sunburst frame who hangs above my stove. From deep inside, the voice of my grandmother spoke. She was a western pioneer of a civilizing kind seldom represented in the movies. Fading strawberry-blond hair piled elegantly on her head, Grandmama knew how to ride sidesaddle, to make peach chutney, and to pronounce "Mama" properly, with the accent on the final syllable. "Joan," she said, "modulate your voice. I can't understand you when you shriek." The water flowed steady into the sink, the soap suds crept between my fingers, the world's order was unchanged. I modulated my inner voice and wondered what to do.

The phone rang. It was the pediatrician's office. Apparently Rick had an appointment with them scheduled after the EEG. Since there was no EEG he had thought he could let it go by. I relayed this to the nurse on the phone, she relayed it to the doctor and the word came back—we were supposed to go in anyway. They wanted to see Ned.

Rick and I woke and dressed our sleepy boy and drove him to the doctors' office. The nurse on the phone had indicated that our regular doctor, Dr. Johnson, was not there, but it did not matter to me much. The man seemed perfectly capable of treating my children's ear infections and staying on top of routine injections but I had never particularly liked him.

When we arrived we were shown into a small examining room. Rick and I sat side by side in the two straight-backed chairs against the short wall; Ned exposed the bottoms of his feet to us as he lay on the examining table along the long one. A desk, with various neutral medical wares upon it, occupied the other long wall; there was a wheeled stool on which the doctor could presumably scoot from table to desk. A vapid poster about childhood occupied the facing short wall, which Rick and I contemplated while Ned snoozed.

After about ten minutes a tall, lanky man with sandy blond hair and a friendly manner arrived. "Hi," he said. "I'm Dr. Lyman." He looked at Ned, who was almost asleep, and grinned.

How are you, young man?" he asked. Ned grinned back. "That's quite an egg you've got there," he observed of Ned's bruise. "Does it hurt?"

"Only if you press on it," Ned replied, proudly fingering the lump.

Dr. Lyman began a standard checkup. He looked into Ned's eyes and his ears. He pulled up Ned's shirt to listen to his heart and lungs.

"Do you want these?" he asked of the electrodes still stuck to Ned's chest.

"Oh, yes!" Ned answered proudly. "My friends will want to see them."

"You look like the bionic man," Dr. Lyman said, and he cheerfully listened to Ned's chest around the strange attachments. He then moved into a number of simple neurological tests. He had Ned walk a straight line, checked his reflexes, and checked his peripheral vision. All seemed perfectly normal. "Well," he said finally, "you're certainly healthy! How do you feel?"

"Tired," Ned responded and lay comfortably back down on the examining table.

"He looks fine," Dr. Lyman said, turning to us. "How are you?"

The question was electrifying. Until it was asked, although Rick and I were deeply involved in the situation, we had had no acknowledged role at all. We were simply "the responsible adults," charged with being sure that directions were followed. Rick poured out his story. Dr. Lyman listened quietly, his upper body draped on the desk, his long torso and legs un-self-consciously moving a little on the wheeled three-legged stool. When Rick was done, Dr. Lyman sat up. "You have just had the worst experience that can ever happen to a parent," he said gravely. "There is nothing more frightening than seeing your child in seizure."

They looked at each other for a moment. Then the doctor broke the spell. "So, . . . you've done it all!" he said with a broad smile. Rick visibly relaxed, and smiled back.

In the next fifteen minutes Dr. Lyman explained that what Ned had experienced, a period of about five minutes of convulsions followed by forty-five minutes of unconsciousness, followed by vomiting, exhaustion, and then his usual state was "normal" insofar as any seizure could be described as normal. The treatment for such seizures was simply commonsense—to clear the area of things like table legs so Ned would not hurt himself as he flailed about, and simply wait until the seizure was over. Unless convulsions last longer than five minutes, an episode of seizure might not even require a doctor to be called. As for the causes, most seizures are idiopathic—no specific cause is ever known, they are just part of an individual's makeup. Others have clear causes that can be found in the brain, but Dr. Lyman did not see any reason to put Ned into this category. We would, of course, follow through with more precise tests, but at the moment it was striking that Ned displayed none of the other neurological symptoms one would expect if there was a tumor or something like that.

"What about Ned now?" I asked. "Do we need to watch over him tonight? What do we do tomorrow? When is it safe to send him back to school?"

"What about Ned now?" the doctor echoed. "He looks fine to me! Are you fine, Ned?" The doctor grinned at the positive response. "He can certainly go back to school tomorrow. The good thing about a seizure is that when its over, it's over."

Rick and I left the building with Ned, so impressed by Dr. Lyman that we agreed to change pediatricians so Ned would be under his care. We took the privilege of frantic parents, and had negotiated the switch in doctors within the week.

Professional

"The good thing about a seizure is that when it's over, it's over." Dr. Lyman's observation became Ned's and my motto for the ensuing months. His first and only grand mal was a devastating performance, but by the time I saw him, five hours later, he was tired, but otherwise perfectly normal. The next morning he was in school again, the only physical reminder of the previous day's drama being the large "egg" on his head, and the metallic stickers he so proudly displayed. Not that anyone needed a reminder; everyone who had been there had been shaken to the very core. Ned, who had been unconscious for the entire episode, was unprepared for the concerned solicitude his appearance provoked in everyone from janitor to principal. Overnight Dr. Lyman's reassurance was transmogrified into expertise and I spent several hours explaining the fine points of convulsive seizures to a variety of those who were working with Ned.

Explanations were required on another level as well. Many of his friends had spent their evenings telling their parents about Ned's performance: "Ned had to go to the hospital in an ambulance. He was fooling around after lunch and crawled under the table. Mrs. Black and Mr. Rogers lifted it up to make him come out, but they dropped it on him and knocked him out. Mr. Kerry *ran* in the lunchroom!" Dr. Gasparian's exercise in interviewing those who were with Ned proved useful as a way to combat the urban legend that was fast forming among the elementary school set.

The shock and concern were real, but there is no room for sustained personal drama either in a large public school or in the press of middle-class life. By ten o'clock I was home, alone, and at loose ends. It was too late to catch the train to Boston. I called the Dibner Institute to cancel a lunch appointment, but there was a larger issue as well. I had to ask about my seminar.

The weekly Tuesday seminars are the heart of the communal life at the Dibner Institute. At these events the fellows present works-in-progress to the other fellows as well as to invited guests from the

11

Greater Boston Area. The seminars give fellows a chance to interest others in what they are doing, and to invite responses, new ideas, suggestions. They are the central event of the fellowship year. Mine was scheduled for the Tuesday before Thanksgiving, not even two weeks away.

The weeks before a seminar are a period of intense work. During the months of September and October I had read a great deal and focused my thinking about Victorian probability theory. At the beginning of November it was time to begin writing. But this new development with Ned, was threatening my time. I was not sure I would be able to put together a strong presentation while I was straightening out whatever his problem was. I asked whether my seminar could be postponed.

"But the schedule is all planned! Your seminar's on the fall poster and we've already sent flyers to Harvard, BU, MIT, and Northeastern. It would be just too complicated to change it now."

I paused on my end of the line.

"You're a professional! I know you can do it."

Yes, of course I could do it.

I found myself thinking about Grandmama, who loved to tell us tales of life in a log cabin in Lewiston, Idaho. They tended to be more morality tale than strict autobiography; people were bigger, stronger, and somehow more good in the days when she rode with her father through the Bitterroots. Her mother bore five boys and one girl, but Grandmama was the only one who survived past the age of two. She told of killing, plucking, and cooking chickens for her grieving mother while her lawyer father was riding the circuit.

The world that bloomed in Grandmama's tales was determinedly literate and Anglophilic. The cabin she described was spotless. In the frigid winters, she and her parents huddled around the stove reading Shakespeare, Sir Walter Scott, Alfred Lord Tennyson and, of course, the King James Bible. In the hot summers, the little cherub, now hanging in my kitchen, was used to cover the unsightly round hole left by the removal of the stove.

Grandmama was not all stories. She was a very real presence in my childhood. I first really noticed her when I was eight. Until then I had lived with my three siblings—an older sister and two younger brothers— in the Boston area where Daddy was in graduate school. But then we moved to Seattle, where Daddy had a job and Mummy had a sister. When we visited Grandmama and Grandad in Portland, Oregon, Grandad cracked walnuts for us; Grandmama made sure we sat up straight and drank all of our milk.

Grandad was killed by a car one Friday night that year. Robert, Peter, and I stood in the hall and listened to Mummy crying in her bedroom. I tried to explain: "He was her father, you know." We were fearfully quiet and good for Daddy when she went to Portland for the funeral.

A few weeks later, Grandmama came to visit. "Your grandfather was a real gentleman, Joan," she said. "I want you to memorize the fifteenth psalm for him."

Lord, who shall abide in thy tabernacle? who shall dwell in thy holy hill?
He that walketh uprightly, and worketh righteousness, and speaketh the truth in his heart.
He that backbiteth not with his tongue, nor doeth evil to his neighbour, nor taketh up a reproach against his neighbour.
In whose eyes a vile person is contemned; but he honoureth them that fear the Lord. He that sweareth to his own hurt, and changeth not.
He that putteth not out his money to usury, nor taketh reward against the innocent. He that doeth these things shall never be moved.

Mummy had responded to Grandmama's strict Episcopal upbringing by becoming a determined Unitarian, but Grandmama's committed religiosity was very powerful. "How can I please God?" I asked her after she had explained the meanings of "backbite," "usury," and "sweareth to his own hurt."

"You can help your mother," she said. "Next year she will begin teaching in Barbara's school. It is far away and she will have to leave early in the morning. You can make breakfast and then clean up after she and Barbara have gone. Robert and Peter are younger than you. You can make sure they are properly dressed and get to school on time. On Tuesdays and Fridays you can make the bread and set it out to rise before you go. When you get home from school you can knead and bake it before dinner."

On Saturday Grandmama went back to Portland. "I have my Sunday school class to teach. I never miss it. Reverend Millman offered to have someone else come the Sunday after Grandad was killed, but I did not let him. What kind of example would I have set for those young people, not coming to our class because of a personal sadness?"

Throughout elementary school, I faithfully followed Grandmama's direction through morning after morning of breakfasts: boiled eggs with toast, hot cereal, muffins, or pancakes. On Tuesdays and Fridays we usually had cold cereal so I had time to make the bread, six loaves at a time in the hand-cranked pail. After the dishes Robert, Peter, and I went off to school. Together we devised schemes to keep Billy, our beagle, from either howling or following us.

After school the boys and I came home together, a tight little group. We did not have many friends; at that time we were newcomers to Seattle, and easterners, and were unique in having a working mother. "If you accept hospitality, it must be returned, and you can't have friends over when I'm not here, Joan," Mummy told me. It did not really matter, though. The three of us were quite content with each other. I punched Steve Johnson, when he called Peter "four-eyes." I made malted milks for Robert because he was too skinny. We played rollicking games of tag, of hide and seek, of "Witchy," the details of which I can't remember. We practiced the piano; at some point we formed a club in which we knitted strange little baby things that we donated to the Orthopedic Hospital. Mummy was always home by five, if not earlier, to listen to our days and make dinner.

In the evenings I found Grandmama's world in the books that I read: *Little House in the Big Woods, Rebecca of Sunnybrook Farm, Little Men, What Katy Did, Waterbabies, The Fairchild Family, The Swiss Family Robinson.* In the midst of my family, Laurelhurst Elementary School, and the Unitarian church, I lived my version of a Victorian childhood: comfortable, disciplined, and supported by a gentlemanly God.

"You're a professional!" The response called me back to that warm world of discipline and order. Ned had had a strange experience, but everyone seemed to agree that now he was fine. There was no excuse for me to crumble into some kind of self-indulgent lassitude because of baseless fears. I hadn't planned to be at home, but I did have a biography of a nineteenth-century mathematician, Augustus De Morgan, that I'd brought as reading for the train. So, I turned on the heat in the apartment, made a batch of bread, and curled up with a Victorian book.

In mathematics, De Morgan is a rather idiosyncratic figure known for a number of bits and pieces. Perhaps his most well-known contribution is the "four-color problem":

A student of mine asked me to-day to give him a reason for a fact which I did not know was a fact, and do not yet. He says, that if a figure be anyhow divided, and the compartments differently coloured, so that figures with any portion of common boundary *line* are differently coloured—four colours may be wanted, but not more. Query cannot a necessity for five or more be invented?

De Morgan shared this problem with a number of correspondents, none of whom was particularly interested: "I am not likely to attempt your 'quaternion of colours' very soon." De Morgan, however, chewed on it for several years. He went around and around about whether it was true and, if so, what it was based on.

After his death, De Morgan's conjecture was picked up by another British mathematician who made it public. This time it "took," and attempts to prove it engaged a great deal of mathematical energy. It was finally confirmed in the 1970s by a computer that cranked for hours checking every possible permutation and combination.

But the computer's feat has just generated more discussion about what it might mean to say that a computer had "proved" a theorem: Web sites go on and on about it. All of which would have thrilled De Morgan. He loved nothing more than mathematical puzzles and convoluted discussions about the nature of mathematics, of proof, of logic. He was part of my seminar paper because he was one of the first people to write about probability theory in England.

The biography of De Morgan I was reading was a laudatory piece, written soon after he died in 1871, by his wife, Sophia. She related how he was born in India in 1806, the fifth child born to an English lieutenant colonel. His family brought him back to England when he was seven months old, but not before he had lost the sight of his right eye to what he variously called "sore-eye," or "opthamalia." [I suspect traucoma.] His father died when he was ten, but the colonel left his wife with the wherewithal to care for their four surviving children. Perhaps because he was partially blind, the young De Morgan seems always to have been quiet and studious in school. In the book, De Morgan's wife struggled to show that from early on he was particularly interested in mathematics, but I was not entirely convinced.

In any case, De Morgan entered Trinity College, Cambridge, at the then-normal age of sixteen, and received his degree in the expected three years' time. He did very well, finishing fourth in his class, but he did not stay to pursue his studies further. Cambridge was an Anglican institution, and the young De Morgan was unwilling to subscribe to the thirty-nine articles of the creed. So he went back to London.

London in the 1820s was a happening place. The industrial revolution was just beginning to make itself felt, business was beginning to boom, and a new group of people were on the way up. The Church of England was the church of the aristocracy, but many of those in the rising middle class were dissenters: Methodists, Quakers, Unitarians, even

Jews. The young De Morgan, who had refused to conform in Cambridge, fit in beautifully.

At Cambridge, De Morgan had considered medicine as a career, but an old friend persuaded him that "he was not pliant enough, and could not, or would not, be sufficiently ready to adapt himself to the fancies and peculiarities he would meet with to make him a popular doctor." From half a century's distance, Sophia loyally disagreed: "Had he been a physician, his fanciful and self-tormenting patients would have thought him the worst of their ills, his milder cases of real suffering would have been cheered by his bantering kindness, while severe and dangerous malady would have felt the presence of the sympathy which money cannot buy, shown with a delicacy which benevolence itself cannot always command."

Whatever might have been his proclivities for medicine, De Morgan set out to study for the bar. He was not a happy barrister, though; he much preferred mathematics. Whenever he could get away, he hung out at the office of the Nautical Almanac, where he came to know William Frend, a London mathematician and religious radical. The two got along famously, and the young man began to spend his evenings in Frend's household. It is there that De Morgan met his future wife, Frend's daughter, Sophia.

Sophia related: "He then looked so much older than he was that we were surprised by hearing his real age—just twenty-one. I was nineteen. We soon found out that this 'rising man,' of whom great things were expected in science, and who had evidently read so much, could rival us in love of fun, fairy tales, and ghost stories, and even showed me a new figure in CAT's cradle. . . . His hair and whiskers were very thick and curly; he was not bald till thirty years after."

Among other things, Frend was deeply involved in founding the London University (later University College) in reaction to the Anglican constraints of Cambridge and Oxford. The new institution was supported by "the great body of enlightened Jews and Dissenters, held back by religious tests from sharing in University advantages, but intelligent enough to perceive the value of what they lost and rich enough to supply the want for themselves." With Frend's support, at the age of twenty-one, De Morgan landed the position as mathematics professor in this brand-new secular university.

At his new job, De Morgan pioneered the divided life of the academic professional, leaving his religion at home during his long days at work. The university was nonresidential so that the students could lead a divided life as well: supported in their religion at home, independent of it at the university. We have become so used to this separation that it is tempting to forget how serious a cleavage it was in an age when religion, or lack thereof, was a major defining force of everyone's life.

But De Morgan had no trouble keeping his religion, whatever it was, to himself. He was a preeminently rational young man who found his mind adequate to the complexities of the world around him. In social situations he tended to be more wry observer than participant: "I once saw him stand by, with a half-amused half-interested look, while a discussion was going on between two learned professors on matter and spirit, the future life, and a Creator . . . without uttering a word. When I asked him what he thought of the arguments, he said, 'I don't understand them, but then I'm not a philosopher.' Then he repeated laughingly to himself a few words uttered by one of the speakers, and said, 'Poor _____, he does not see that if what he said were true, he would not be here to say it."

At home with the Frends, De Morgan was more engaged. He played flute duets with one of Sophia's sisters. "He liked puzzles about numbers, as he liked riddles, and, when *very good*, plays upon words and puns." This interest in strange twists of words and their meanings made sense to me from what I knew of De Morgan's mathematics. At the time he was involved in algebra. He was looking at equations like $(a^2 - b^2) = (a + b)(a - b)$ wondering what it means to say that this bunch of symbols is "true." Do a and b have to be numbers? Could they refer to geometrical lines? to absolutely anything that fit the form? De Morgan ultimately decided that their truth might refer to anything that fit the form, but it took him some time to come to this conclusion. "At first it seemed to us something like symbols bewitched and running around the world in search of meaning."

There were ups and downs in De Morgan's early years in London. The new university was a fractious place and he soon resigned in protest because he believed religion had entered into a hiring decision. For a while he supported himself with writing and working for an insurance company. But he never doubted himself or the rational world he lived in, and after a couple of years he renegotiated his position at the university to resume the teaching he loved.

In 1836, however, De Morgan received a rude shock. His sister died during childbirth, leaving an infant son and three little girls behind. De Morgan was devastated. Even he could not make sense of the death of someone so beloved, so healthy, and so needed. Within a year he and Sophia were married and she was pregnant with the first of what were to be seven children. I was warmed by this response on the part of a grieving brother.

It was also at this point that the biography became relevant to my seminar. De Morgan wrote about probability theory in the first year of his marriage to Sophia. It was an interesting connection. I had always seen probability theory as an obvious object for De Morgan's interest because of its ties to insurance. Certainly this was a major part of its hold on him, and he addressed a small book directly to insurance issues. But the timing of his interest suggested to me the importance of another approach to the theory. "The word *probable*," De Morgan wrote in the year he married Sophia, "as commonly applied to a coming event, indicates many different degrees of that feeling with which the mind looks at the prospects of the future, and which depends upon the habits derived from looking at the past."

This was a strikingly personal definition of probability, but De Morgan immediately moved to temper its private aspects. In a subsequent paragraph he made a distinction between what he labeled *moral probability*, which "depended upon the constitution of the individual, his knowledge of the circumstances and the effect the event will produce," and *mathematical probability*, in which the individual "is disposed to consider equal successive changes of favourable circumstances into unfavourable, or *vice versâ*, as of equal importance." He then summarily dumped the personal view: "In the future," he clarified, "*probability* means *mathematical probability*, unless the contrary be specified."

Late in the 1830s Charles Darwin was weighing his decision to marry with a list of pros: "Charms of music & female chit chat." and cons: "Loss of time.—cannot read in the evenings." Somewhere in the same city De Morgan was adding mathematical precision to the exercise by calculating specific risks. Both men decided to get married, but, whatever they might say, I doubted whether it was really on the basis of a rational calculation.

"Hey, Mom! I'm home!"

Ned sounded cheery. He looked well. I put down De Morgan. My boy wiggled as I hugged him and snuffled his hair.

Mild Abnormality, Both Sides

At first things seemed remarkably easy on Friday when Ned and I returned to Dr. Gasparian for his EEG, or electroencephalogram, a procedure to show brain waves. A nurse took him out of Dr. Gasparian's waiting room, explaining to me that the test was painless but long—about an hour. During it Ned was to lie completely still in a darkened room thinking about as little as possible; distractions, including mothers, were to be avoided at all costs. I accepted her explanation and retired to read banal magazines in the waiting room.

Four ancient issues of *People* later, Ned reappeared, a bit sleepy from enforced rest but otherwise unscathed. Soon thereafter Dr. Gasparian called us into his small office. He had a folded computer printout about the size of a small urban telephone book on which was a series of jagged curves. While we sat there he flipped through its pages, once, twice, and then again, slowing a bit here and there. Then he pronounced: "Mild abnormality, both sides."

"What does that mean?" I tried after a brief pause.

"Well, it could be just the aftermath of the seizure or it could be something else. It is very slight. But, since he has had previous episodes we should probably put him on a medication. He could take Dilantin, Tegretol, or phenobarbital. Which do you want?"

"I don't know. Does he have to go on medication?"

"You don't want him to have another seizure, do you?"

"No."

"Well, which do you want?"

"Are these mind-altering drugs?"

"I guess you could say that. They are to try to stop seizures in the brain, after all. Children usually get used to them, though."

"What are the differences?"

"Well, mothers don't usually like phenobarbital because it tends to reduce school performance. Dilantin causes problems for your teeth. Tegretol sometimes affects liver function or lowers the white blood cell count."

I ruled out phenobarbital. "What happens to your teeth?" I asked.

"They rot," he replied. "But if you brush them a lot, they are sometimes OK."

I thought of Ned's clean, cavityless mouth. "What about your liver?" I asked.

"If there is a problem, you would take him off Tegretol. You just do blood tests to stay on top of it."

"How long would he be on the drug? For the rest of his life?"

"Probably. If he doesn't want seizures."

"Can I decide now and then change my mind after I talk to his father?"

"No. To be effective they have to build up for some time."

I sat for a moment, trapped, not knowing what to do.

"Which do you want?" the doctor asked.

"I don't know. I can't just decide something like this. I have to think about it."

"Well this is Veteran's Day weekend and I am leaving town in a couple of hours. You don't want Ned to have another seizure over the weekend."

I was boxed in and could not budge. "I can't make this kind of decision here and now," I said. "I don't know enough about what is going on."

"I've told you," the man said, exasperated. "You can put him on Dilantin or Tegretol. You know the side effects. Which do you want?"

"I don't know," I said.

"Well, I'll talk to your pediatrician," he said.

By the time we got home it was five o'clock. I called Rick at work and explained what I had not done. He was as concerned as I about so precipitously putting Ned on a lifetime of medication. "We'll talk it over with Dr. Lyman," he promised.

I turned my attention to dinner. The phone rang.

"Hello, Mrs. Richards. This is Dr. Johnson. Dr. Lyman is out of the office but I just took a call from Dr. Gasparian. We need to know whether you want to put Ned on Tegretol or Dilantin."

"I don't know," I said. "What do you think?"

"Well, one or the other," he said.

"Do I have to decide right now?" I said as the water for the pasta started to boil. "My husband is not here and I want to talk it over with him."

"I am just on my way out of the office," he said. "It is Veteran's Day weekend and my family is going out of town."

I had never seen Veteran's Day as a major holiday, but suddenly it loomed large. "Does it matter so much? What are the issues? Can't we think it over and decide on Tuesday?"

"Dr. Gasparian thinks Ned should be on something. I would just like to write the prescription before I go. Which do you want?"

I did not scream, but I did not answer his question either. "I cannot make this kind of decision under these circumstances," I said, hung up the phone, and dumped the pasta into the water.

That night I broke an ironclad rule and talked things over with two of my medical friends. Slowly, patiently, they explained that it was important that Ned be on a medication because seizures pattern themselves in your brain: it is harder to stop a series than to stop a single one. The one Ned had just had raised the probabilities of his having another, enormously. If we were to allow a second, the probability of a third would be even greater. The seizures had to be stopped now. As for the drugs, the choice was to a large extent academic. My friends leaned towards Tegretol, but did not think it mattered particularly which he was on. There might be a bit of an adjustment period, but within a couple of weeks it seemed Ned would not notice the effects at all. After I had conversations with my medical friends, Rick had to have his conversations with his—he needed to be clear as much as I. After two hours on the phones we were both reconciled to the reality that faced us. We got a prescription from the pediatrician on call and gave Ned his first dose of Tegretol after breakfast on Saturday morning.

The second part of Dr. Gasparian's pronouncement, "both sides," referred to the location of the abnormality in Ned's brain waves. In a telephone call on Wednesday, Dr. Lyman found the observation that it seemed to come from both sides of the brain to be reassuring. The lack of specificity suggested that the cause of the seizure might fit into his catchall category of "idiopathic" as opposed to some localized problem. The question was important enough that the pediatrician pushed the diagnostic process another step. I was glad for his decision to be cautious and send us to a radiologist who could take a picture of the internal structure of Ned's brain using magnetic resonance imaging, or MRI. The pictures taken with this new and highly refined technology might show something that could be identified as the cause for Ned's seizures.

The radiologist's secretary was somewhat apprehensive about working with Ned. When she heard he was only nine and we were talking about an MRI of his brain, she wondered whether we should sedate him. "He will have to lie absolutely still for about an hour in a tube. It makes a lot of noise. Is he a placid child?"

"No, I wouldn't describe him as placid."

"Well nine may be old enough. Perhaps you could bring a tape of music that he likes. He can listen with earphones in the tube."

A tape seemed like a better idea than a sedative, so when the boys got home from school I sent them out to get one. "Get something quiet, Brady. I don't want him bopping out of the tube!"

I watched them to the end of the street. They were such a wonderful pair, alike in their dishwater-blond hair but almost nothing else: Brady such a scholar, Ned such an imp. Ned was a bit tall for his age, but not tall the way Brady was tall. On the doctor's charts Ned hovered at the seventy-fifth percentile in both height and weight, whereas Brady combined the ninetieth percentile of height with the twentieth of weight. In the past two years Brady had shot up; now the difference between them was more than a foot. As they disappeared around the corner, deep in conversation about musical preferences, Ned was taking two dancing steps to each of Brady's long, purposeful strides.

They returned gleeful, and repaired to Brady's room to listen to their treasure. It was not what I would have described as soothing.

"Oh, Mom, it's great! It's R.E.M.! It's *Monster!*" Ned's brown eyes twinkled happily.

From behind his glasses Brady's gray-green ones reached to reassure me. "It's really OK, Mom. It's not heavy metal. And it doesn't have any bad words or anything."

It was dark and pouring rain when Ned and I went searching for the radiologist's office on a decaying commercial strip. I cruised past Blackstone Subaru, Burger King, Tasca Lincoln-Mercury. I squinted at Marshall's, Bed and Bath, Visioncare.

"Oh, Mom! There's a game store! Can we see whether they have *Magic* cards?"

"No, Ned!" I snapped as we passed Academy Swimming Pools for the second time.

"That says MRI," Ned pointed, subdued. I jerked the car sharply into the small, unlit parking lot.

As I had been warned, the test itself was somewhat formidable. Ned and I had first to remove anything with even the possibility of a trace of magnetic material. Then Ned gave his tape to the technician and we went into the room that housed the machine. The machine itself was a massive structure with a tube through it; Ned lay on a trolley outside of the tube. The technician positioned headphones on his ears among the various plastic devices designed to hold his head absolutely still. The whole was then rolled into the tube with strict instructions not to move at all—not even to swallow or blink his eyes. From where I sat next to the apparatus all I could see were Ned's feet in their battered tennis shoes.

The technician then retired to a room behind a glass wall where she could talk to Ned through his earphones. There was a minor crisis when she realized that she had totally erased his precious tape by bringing it into the room with the machine. Ned was not too concerned; he cheerfully asked to be tuned to a rock station that Brady listened to a lot. After the volume had been adjusted, she proceeded to the test.

"The first picture will be four minutes," she said. "Don't forget, it's noisy. And don't forget you must stay still, absolutely still."

"OK," Ned's voice came muffled from the tube.

There was silence while the technician adjusted. Then the machine began to bang—it sounded rather like a distant jackhammer. On and on it banged. It created rhythms in my mind. "You must pay the rent. You must pay the rent. I can't pay the rent. I can't pay the rent. What will they find? What will they find? Will Ned be dead? No, Ned's not dead. No, Ned's not dead." I struggled to clear my mind. "Do keep your cool. Do keep your cool. Do keep your cool." Finally the banging stopped. I could hear the secondhand jangle of Ned's earphone music in the silent room.

"Good job, Ned," said the technician's voice.

I reached over to squeeze a protruding tennis shoe. Ned moved his foot in response. "Don't move, Ned," the voice said. The machine whirred in an adjustment kind of way. Different lights flashed on and off.

"The next picture will take eight minutes," the voice said.

Ned's MRI was on the Friday before Thanksgiving. Dr. Lyman said it might take some time to get back to us about it, but he promised to call before the holiday.

Monday we celebrated Brady's fifteenth birthday—steak, baked potatoes, salad, chocolate cake.

Tuesday was my seminar. De Morgan nodded approvingly as I gave Ned his Tegretol, sent him to school, and caught the Boston train. For two weeks De Morgan's spirit had stood by me as I juggled days and my laptop through Ned's scheduled appointments. Now he cheered me on as I dashed through my morning preparing overheads. His spirit stood by me as I faced the Dibner seminar room and delivered my paper:

In De Morgan's view we all live our lives as gamblers, because we are always moving into an unknown future. In all of our thinking we are constantly betting on unknown outcomes. In all cases we are thinking probabilistically.

Wednesday, as I was preparing dinner, the phone rang.

"Hello, Mrs. Richards. This is Dr. Lyman. There seems to be a spot on Ned's MRI. It is small and may well be nothing, perhaps the scar of an old injury or something like that . . ."—Ned was about six when he flew over his handlebars onto the curb. I saw again the dent in his helmet.—". . . but we need to find out what it is. We have to get another set of pictures, this time with contrast, to see whether it is growing tissue or not. This time they will inject Ned with a dye; it will make the lesion light up if it is living tissue. The radiologist's schedule was full, but this is important. He has scheduled Ned after hours, Friday afternoon at five o'clock." Growing tissue? Living tissue? A brain tumor? Ned could have a brain tumor? There was no public or private here; no determined display of confident effectiveness.

"Thank you," I said, preternaturally calm. "We will be there."

Thursday was Thanksgiving. We spent it with my great Aunt Priscilla. She was an East Coast aunt, on my father's side, no relation of Grandmama. She had been a dear friend to Rick and me for more than twenty-five years. We were married in her house.

I hugged her gently. At ninety-four she had shrunk to the size of a bird, and I almost feared breaking her bones.

"How are you?" she asked brightly. "And how are the boys?"

"We couldn't be better!" I yelled.

"Yes, the weather has been lovely," she replied. Virtually blind and deaf, Aunt Priscilla lived behind a thick wall of sensory deprivation. Communication was always rather one-sided.

While I moved around her familiar kitchen preparing a traditional Thanksgiving dinner, Rick patiently followed Aunt Priscilla's lead through a bewildering ritual of formal table setting. "Oh, Rick! We need the good silver. . . . You put the salad forks on the outside and then the dinner forks . . . No, Rick! Those are the dessert forks! They go on the top next to the dessert spoons. . . . Yes, that's good. The flowered china." The boys watched television and drank ginger ale.

At dinner we all followed Aunt Priscilla's conversational lead. She moved from one to the other of us, going through her standard list of questions about our work, our studies, our play. Many times I have found the approach frustrating but on this blank day between MRI reports it was a great relief. She could hear so little that our answers didn't matter a great deal, but we threw ourselves into the process. Momentarily safe, our family "gathered together to ask the Lord's blessing."

The next afternoon Rick and I both went with Ned for the MRI with contrast. Within an hour of our returning home the phone rang.

"Hello, Mrs. Richards." Dr. Lyman did not sound his cheery self. "It appears that the lesion is 'hot,'" he said.

"What does that mean?"

"It means that the lesion is some kind of living tissue. I can't tell you anything more than that. I don't know enough about how to read this kind of picture."

I stayed frozen and calm. "OK, then. But what do we do?"

"On Monday I am going to make an appointment for you to talk to Dr. Harlow. He is a neurosurgeon here in town. He is good with children."

My boys were both bald babies. I loved the feel of their downy skulls, crowned by a throbbing soft spot. I'd cup it protectively with my palm. Inside their brains were growing.

Then, one day, their hair flashed forth, all at once, each strand the same length. For two weeks, three weeks, their skulls were surrounded with an aura of astonished dandelion fluff. It would lean away if I blew on it, and leap back when I stopped. I could brush it with my hand and never touch the gleaming, throbbing skull beneath.

And then, as suddenly as it had come, the aura was gone. The fluff became hair and lay down. Their skulls disappeared and they became little boys. But I always knew their skulls were there, under the vagaries of haircuts and dirt. I could sniff them out after a bath.

"Will my skull still be strong after they cut it?" Ned asked.

"Of course," I reassured him, but I was lying. I did not know.

My freeze was so deep I could barely function. "Get yourself a notebook," my sister Barbara advised over the phone. "Write down your questions so you don't forget them. Write down Ned's too."

I found on my desk a small yellow spiral notebook, and carefully wrote Ned's only question on the first page. "Will my skull still be strong after they cut it?" I called my brother Robert, who is a radiologist, to find out what questions I should ask. Dutifully I wrote them down on the next page: "Is the lesion on the right or the left side?" "How large is it?" "Is it on the surface?" "If not, where is it?" Then I added mine to the list. "What kind of incision will you make?" "How long will the operation take?" "How long will Ned be in the hospital?"

Technically, Dr. Harlow was not a pediatric neurosurgeon. What recommended him was that he was the father of young children and saw the world as a parent. At Dr. Lyman's request, Dr. Harlow took time from his lunch on Tuesday so we would not be left in limbo longer than was necessary. At noon, Rick, Ned, and I trembled into his office with Ned's MRI pictures.

The surgeon arranged the MRI pictures on a lighted reader. It was shocking to see an image of Ned's brain, his eyes on stalks. Even in the split second before I turned resolutely away I could see the lesion shining brightly on the left side. "Hmm . . ." Dr. Harlow mumbled, looking closely at the pictures. "There is certainly something there. I believe it is a meningioma: that would mean that it is benign. . . . It may not grow at all. I would not want to blind your child to take out something that will not grow. . . . It is certainly very small. I would not want to go in and be unable to find it. From a neurosurgical point of view I would say it is not worth an operation."

I carefully wrote down Dr. Harlow's diagnosis on the third page of the little yellow spiral notebook. "Left side, close to occipital lobe, ~1 cm in diameter, ~3 cm deep." All of my questions were irrelevant. The notebook's cover boasted that it contained sixty pages, but it seemed that three would suffice. Dr. Harlow said it was benign and we could let it be. Ned was disappointed not to be able to brag to his friends about an operation, but Rick and I could not have been more relieved. We positively danced out of Dr. Harlow's office.

Two days later, as I was preparing dinner, the telephone rang.

"Hello, Mrs. Richards. This is Dr. Gasparian. I have talked to Dr. Harlow, and he does not think an operation is in order. You should know, though, that as Ned's neurologist, I believe that the lesion is what is causing his seizures. Dr. Bentley is a very important seizure surgeon from Yale. He will be here next week for a conference. I would like to present Ned's case at that time. Would you be willing to bring him and the MRI pictures to the hospital next Wednesday morning? Dr. Bentley and others will want to talk to him for a little bit about his seizures and headaches but it will be only about fifteen minutes. Then you can go home."

I didn't particularly like Dr. Gasparian, and I had no intention of letting his dreariness prevail over Dr. Harlow's good sense. Still I knew that it is important for doctors to learn as much as they can from cases like Ned's. I was happy to let our close call educate a conference of neurosurgeons.

At eight-thirty on Wednesday morning Ned, Rick, and I made our way through the unfamiliar halls of the hospital looking for the neurology conference in the Eddy Auditorium.

"Well, where's the Neddy Auditorium?" Rick asked, scanning the informational signs.

"Over here, Dad."

"No, that's not it. That's the Eddy Auditorium."

"That's what we want, Dad."

"No it's not. It's *you* who is supposed to be going to this place, isn't it? You're not Eddy, you're Neddy. We need the Neddy Auditorium."

"Don't be silly, Dad!"

"Silly? Who's silly?"

"*You're* silly, Dad!"

"OK! OK! Have it your way! We'll go to the Eddy Auditorium. All those doctors in the Neddy Auditorium are going to be sad, though."

"Dad!"

"Ned!"

"Enough you guys," I said as we came to the open space by the doors of the auditorium.

Dr. Gasparian was there, bustling busily about, orchestrating his presentation. "Elizabeth, you will go first," he said to a lanky girl of about twelve, who was waiting with her mother. "Dr. Bentley will ask you a couple of questions about your seizures. Maybe some of the other doctors will too. It won't be long. I'll be there and so will your mother. It's nothing to worry about."

Elizabeth smiled shyly. Her teeth were covered with braces. "OK," she said.

Dr. Gasparian turned to Ned. "I'll come get you when Dr. Bentley is ready. It might be a little while after Elizabeth comes out. Just wait out here until I come. Don't go in until I say to."

"OK," said Ned.

Rick recognized Dr. Harlow among the coffee-drinking medics and went over to talk to him. Ned sat on my lap holding the envelope of MRI pictures; Elizabeth did the same with her mother. The girl's legs reached the ground; Ned's did not. We mothers smiled silently at each other, but conversation was dangerous. I did not want to ask about their situation. Perhaps they had not been as lucky as we had. Nine o'clock came and the doctors moved into the auditorium. Dr. Gasparian called Elizabeth in. About fifteen minutes later it was Ned's turn.

About thirty doctors were sprinkled through the chairs of an auditorium that could have seated three times that number. Ned held Rick's and my hands as Dr. Gasparian led us down the aisle to the stage at the front. Ned stood in front of us as we turned to face the room.

"This is Edward Richards," Dr. Gasparian said. "He is nine years old. He had his first convulsive seizure in the school lunchroom on November 9."

Ned looked out into the dimly lit room. "It's OK, Neddy," I whispered from behind.

"Well, Edward," said a man seated in the front row. I guessed it was Dr. Bentley. "Can you tell us about your seizure?"

"No!" Ned said.

The doctor was a bit startled. "Why not?" he asked.

"Well, you see," said Ned informatively, "when you have a seizure you don't remember it. You move and everything—I banged my head on the table—but then you don't remember it at all. That's the way it is with seizures."

A collective chuckle arose from the audience and Dr. Bentley smiled. "I see," he said. "Can you tell me the last thing you *do* remember? *before* the seizure?"

Ned thought for a moment. "I saw the pool table," he said.

"The pool table?"

"The pool table."

"Is there a pool table in your school lunchroom?"

"No, but I saw one."

"Did you see its legs?" the doctor tried.

"No," Ned replied. "It was the top of the table."

"Did it have pockets?"

"No, it was the middle."

"Were there balls on the table?"

"No, no one was playing."

"How did you know it was a pool table, then?"

"It was green!" Ned said.

Again the doctors laughed. Ned was in his element performing before a rapt audience. He beamed his way down the aisle when the questions were over.

"Don't play pool! It's not cool!" Rick said as we went back to the car.

"Dad!" said Ned.

"Don't play pool! Don't be a fool!" Rick tried.

"I'm not a fool! I go to school!" Ned got into the swing as we drove out of the parking lot.

That evening, as I was preparing dinner, Dr. Gasparian called. "Thank you for bringing Ned to the conference," he said. "His case is a very interesting one and we had a good discussion about it. Dr. Harlow still does not think that an operation is in order, but Dr. Bentley is not sure it is a meningioma. He thinks it might be an astrocytoma or a glioma. Dr. Starkey thought . . ."

"Just a moment," I interrupted, my voice strangled. I put down the phone, moving like an automaton to my desk where I found the little yellow notebook and a pencil. Returning to the kitchen, I wrote "Dr. Bentley is not sure it is a meningioma" on the fourth page. I picked up the phone and held it between my shoulder and my ear. "Sorry," I said. "I'm trying to write this down. What did Dr. Bentley think it might be?"

Dr. Gasparian went back to the discussion about Ned's case. There was no problem seeing the lesion. The questions concerned diagnoses and treatment: what it was and what should be done about it. The two were closely related—the more benign the tumor, the less dramatic were the risks surgeons were willing to contemplate to remove it. "Meningioma," "glioma," "astrocytoma," "hamartoma," the terms spilled out from the phone: "tricky location," "deep," "could be a problem," ran the surgeons' opinions.

"Ned, could you please set the table. Now!" I barked at the living son in the next room as I wrote the words and phrases that could be his life sentence in the little yellow spiral notebook.

After about fifteen minutes there seemed to be no new words to utter, no new opinions to pronounce. Dr. Gasparian and his gaggle of interested experts moved on to another problem. I had preserved the jumble of their terms and phrases in the yellow notebook, but they revealed neither conclusion nor clear direction. The following Wednesday, Dr. Lyman cleared some real time at the end of his day so we could talk things over

"All these '-omas?' Oh yes, they usually refer to the kinds of cells involved in the process. So, let's go through these one by one. 'Meningioma.' That arises from the meninges, the covering of the brain. A meningioma is usually very benign. If you can get it out it is just gone. 'Astrocytoma.' That just means it involves astrocytes. They are little cells that look like stars. That's the 'astro' part, like astronomy. Astrocytomas are quite common; there are all different kinds. Some are more of a problem than others. 'Glioma.' Well, gliomas tend to be more aggressive. . . ."

Dr. Lyman warmed to the topic of brain tumors, happily calling up stored expertise little needed in his daily round of ear infections and broken limbs. Dutifully I sat while he explained, trying to keep my concentration fixed by writing what he said in the spiral notebook. I kept my eyes down and my tears silent as with each new terminological challenge he became less able to smooth over the seriousness of the situation that faced Ned. He looked at me expectantly, for the next term to explain.

"Are you crying?" he asked, startled. He recalled himself. "Ah, yes!" he said, a bit chagrined. "You are his mother."

I had been Ned's mother for nine years and it was often difficult. Brady had always seemed so like me, I could easily connect to the intellectual world in which he lived. Ned was not. He was strong-willed, stubborn, and often resistant to my direction. "He's your child, Rick!" I'd cry in despair, when he was particularly wild, did not want to read a book, or would not entertain himself.

"Ah, yes! You are his mother." I found now what that meant. I found Ned entangled in everything I was—my hopes, my fears, my life itself. His smile lifted me on dark days, his boundless self-confidence bolstered me, his resilience became mine. There were others in my family, but none was Ned. There was nothing more important than Ned.

Now Ned was being thrust into a world of doctors who did not see him as Ned. For them he was a sick child, a patient, an interesting case. I needed their help but I could not accept their perspective. In their offices I was trapped in a no-man's land.

Dr. Lyman served as a kind of go-between between Rick and my total engagement and the removed world of the doctors. He was as busy as any of the people we worked with, and we were able to have an actual appointment with him only twice in the entire process. Still he was very important. During these face-to-face meetings and sporadic telephone calls he served as a clearinghouse and translator for the various situations and opinions that precipitated around our son. It was Dr. Lyman who softened the blows of Dr. Gasparian's brusque manner.

The name that arose out of the postconference discussions as the best person to deal with Ned's tumor was Dr. Jennings, and Dr. Lyman's next move was to refer us to him. So, a couple of days after our conversation with Dr. Lyman, I carried the unwieldy envelope containing

Ned's MRIs into the heart of a Boston medical complex. Dr. Jennings's office was in an old and dark part of the building—my route to it lay through back doors, narrow elevators and unmistakable hospital smells. Outside of the office where I dropped off the pictures huddled a drained, pale couple. *Is that what Rick and I look like?* The secretary was on the phone when I arrived, carefully taking notes: "Now, how long was he unconscious? . . . Yes, it is a shock. . . . You say he hit his head when he fell? . . ." I thrust the envelope in her direction and ran. I hoped with all my heart that they would suffice for Dr. Jennings. I did not want to bring Ned into this place—ever.

A few days later Dr. Jennings called Rick at work. "It is too early to tell what this process is," the doctor said. "Wait until the end of March, and then get another set of MRIs. We'll compare them then and decide what to do from there."

Christmas

Our Christmas that year was quiet and, for Rick and me, rather subdued. We did our best with the regular round of neighborhood parties, candlelight services, and general good cheer, but it certainly did not flow from the heart. It had no meaning. "For unto us a child is born"—"For unto us a child is sick," "For unto us a child is threatened"—there was no Christmas in this.

Rick was entangled with his work and could not get time off: "I have a meeting from eight to noon, and a report to finish before a three o'clock appointment. I'll try to be home by five. You'll be all right, won't you, Joan?" I heard the unspoken question behind it: "You'll keep Ned all right, won't you, Joan?" We both knew that I couldn't.

But Ned was fine. Excited by the holiday, he bubbled with schemes for buying presents and pursued ever-more-elaborate cookie recipes. In our midst there *was* a child and he was a fount of life. How could it be that he might die?

Grandmama's voice told me to keep on going as if I understood; as if I saw the way. "God helps those who help themselves." I wanted to hear, but her dutiful directives grated on my inner ear. The spot on Ned's MRI glowed in my mind, a symbol bewitched, searching for meaning in a world of "-*omas*." There were times when getting up at all was a major effort.

Brady was upset by my brittleness. "Come off it, Mom," he said. "The doctors know what they are doing. Ned will be fine." How could I tell him that there are some things even doctors don't know how to handle? Why should I tell him? I knew that it was better to learn from his confidence than to try to bring him to my point of view. I am not fifteen, though, and that kind of faith was hard to muster. The wrenching prayer of another weeping parent rang through my days: "O Lord, I believe. Help now mine unbelief."

A few days after Christmas, Rick was reading to Ned in the living room when he cried out, "It's happening! I'm going to have a seizure!" To us absolutely nothing had happened to change the peaceful moment except for Ned's anguished cry. The room remained warm, light, and cozy. But Ned sat and stared terrified into the room. His concern seemed so utterly unreal I almost said: "Don't be silly. Pull yourself together. There is nothing happening at all!" But I bit back my words. Somewhere deep in Ned's brain something was happening over which he had no control. We had no knowledge of it except what he could tell us. Whatever it was frightened him a great deal. We were frightened as well.

What to do? We did not know. Dr. Lyman had said we should sit Ned on the floor and clear all obstructions from the area if he felt a seizure coming on, but in the event isolating the frightened Ned in that way was an impossible response. I quickly scanned the vicinity for potential obstacles, and moved the coffee table farther from the couch. Then we waited, Rick with Ned on the couch, to see what happened next. Nothing did. After a couple of minutes Ned said it was better. Relieved, but unsure, I said he should go to bed, a suggestion he gratefully accepted. All night I lay with my ear cocked for thumps or bumps that would indicate he was in seizure—there is nothing to say they do not come in the night—but nothing happened. In the morning he was the same as ever. I opened a page in the yellow spiral notebook called "Seizures" and wrote a brief description with the date and time.

A couple of days later we left for a long-planned week of skiing, the high point of our family year. It was always fun to squeeze ourselves into our car and head off, away from all entanglements.Part of the travel ritual involved dinner on the road; we stopped in a rather dreary restaurant in a deserted shopping mall.

"Can I have the steak, Dad? I'm really hungry."

"OK, Brady." Rick was proud of the appetite of his growing son. "Do you want a salad as well?"

"Yes, and fries."

Ned entered the lists: "I want steak too."

"But it's too much for you! Remember last year how you ate too much and it made you sick?" Brady put Ned in his place.

"But I'm bigger than I was last year!"

"You may have a steak if you want," Rick said, supportively.

"Dad! You're spoiling him! Why doesn't anyone in this family make any sense?"

Holding up his hand, Ned gleefully offered the current schoolboy put-down. "Talk to the hand, not to the face! Leave a message after the beep!"

Rick, for his part, held up his hand like a telephone receiver. "Hello? Hello?" he said. "This is a message for Ned. I am going to be skiing the top of the mountain tomorrow afternoon. Are you going to join me?"

"Dad! You're so stupid! I'm going to leave if you guys don't stop being so dumb!"

Never daunted, Rick pressed on. "Oh, Brady! Is that you? I thought I was talking to an answering machine! Are you going to be skiing with me tomorrow morning? Aren't we in the same class?"

"Mom! Tell him to stop! He's being so stupid!"

"Calm down, Brady! It's OK. Cool it, Rick."

And so it went. It was all so normal, but I was not. I was overwhelmed with grief. The "whys" crackled in my head as I looked around at the other people in the room, obliviously eating their meals, their cares normal-sized. My problem was so big, so out of proportion with the bland institutional surroundings and the nondescript clientele; it eclipsed all other thoughts or interaction. I went through the motions of ordering, chatting with the family, eating my meal, but inside I was howling with despair.

A couple came and sat at the table next to us, perching their baby in a high chair. The child was adorable, his head of hair coming in a wild soft mohawk. I resisted with difficulty the temptation to reach out and feel its softness as he smiled only feet away from me. His parents chatted with each other and played with him as they waited to order. I was overwhelmed by the unfairness of the situation. Here they were, with their beloved child. He had no seizures, no brain tumor, no nothing; he was completely fine, his life stretched before him, open and whole. This child was what Ned had been before the seizure exploded in his head. I was overwhelmed with self-pity.

Slowly, it came to me. It was certainly true that the couple's child was just like Ned as a baby, long before he had the slightest hint of a seizure. But the child's healthy infancy did not guarantee his continued health any more than Ned's had his—the present never guarantees the future. I began to see that we had not been singled out by Ned's problems; the fundamental challenge of uncertainty—life and death—is always there. We were just being forced to recognize them. "In the midst of life we are in death," I heard Grandmama's deep, well-modulated voice reading from her prayer book. Knowing this as I did then reduced the gap that fed my self-pity. As dinner ended, I began to rejoin the human race.

❋ ❋ ❋

The baby in the restaurant was only the first step toward my adjustment: the next was on the ski slopes. Before we had left I had plunged telephonically into the world of planning for a "special" child, or whatever was the appropriate term. I tried to locate various organizations for children with seizure disorder for advice as to how to proceed, but ultimately they were less useful than the ski resort itself was. There they had a program to encourage people with a huge range of handicaps to take to the slopes—they were wonderfully willing to help with my thinking about Ned. Finally we settled on a variety of safety measures—a climbing harness with which he could be secured to the chair lift and a helmet. Then we discussed the possibility of my accompanying him in his lesson so that if there were a problem he would be taken care of.

"Oh, no, Mrs. Richards! This is your vacation. We will find a volunteer to ski with him."

Our first morning on the slopes Rick and Brady went skiing together while I bustled around self-importantly, locating the special-needs office, maneuvering Ned into his harness, explaining the basic parameters of the situation to the woman in charge, his ski instructor, and the volunteer who was going to accompany him. They were all calm and relaxed about what I had to say. In particular, his volunteer, who was a nurse getting free skiing for her children in exchange for caring for mine, was totally capable and had no need of my input. "I know seizures," she said cheerily.

Ned stood at her elbow wearing a hat Rick's brother had given him for Christmas. It was multicolored with three unnecessary fingers that either flopped or pointed to the sky. It was weird and fit my impish son perfectly. They got on the chair and he grinned at me as his volunteer snapped him into the chair. The fingers on his hat bobbed as they moved together into the gray day.

I stood until they were out of sight and then wondered what to do. I also had a lesson and a group of people with whom to ski, but under the circumstances it seemed somehow wrong just to head on out. However, standing around quickly lost its charm and skiing seemed the only alternative. So, I got myself suited up and went up the mountain with a couple of my classmates.

"Hi, I'm Susan."

"And I'm Mark."

"Hi, I'm Joan. Are you together?"

"Yes, we got married this time last year. Are you here on your own?"

"No, I'm here with my family. My husband is skiing with my older son. My younger one is with the Ski-Wees."

"How nice! Two boys!"

"Yes, it is nice."

The conversation continued and as the chairlift creaked up the mountain I relaxed into the ways I was like my companions. I also was in desperate need of a vacation. My problems seemed huge, but they were not demanding at the moment. Brady and Rick enjoyed their class together; Ned thrived in his. I threw myself into learning how to ski moguls. If there was a problem with Ned I would certainly hear about it, but in the meantime I could put it down.

The vacation did not wear off. Even as we moved into normal life the peace I had found in the snow stayed with me. Rick went every day to work in the Rhode Island Department of Education. The boys' schools continued unabated. In my Cambridge office I settled down to work. This was a profoundly stabilizing project because I have long found meaning in the history of mathematics; from my college days it has been not only my job but my vocation.

I began to know how special mathematics was amid the confusions of early adolescence. For me the problems began in the sixth grade when I began to grow like a bamboo shoot. By the time I was thirteen I was five feet, nine inches, at least a foot taller than either brother, four inches taller than Barbara, three inches taller than my mother. Throughout junior high school as I struggled to fit the loud, clumsy, fast-growing Joan that I was into the social spaces allotted to young women, mathematics sustained me. In the midst of efforts to maintain my dignity through school dances, clothes shopping, and hair dressing, mathematics provided peace. It was like a daily miracle to hear my classmates read out their answers to problems and find that we had come to the same conclusion. When the rest of life seemed an unending struggle to find the right thing to say, the right place to be, mathematics class was a safe haven. I understood in mathematics class.

Reveling in mathematics was not so straightforward in college, though. Within weeks of my arrival at Harvard I knew there was no place for a girl from a public high school on the West Coast among the competitive and totally self-absorbed men of the mathematics and physics departments. I dabbled sadly in English, history, and French. But I found no meaning there. Then I discovered the history of science. It was Newton who led me in.

I first learned about Newton in physics, because of his theory of gravitation. The beauty of this for me, a homesick freshman, was that the law of gravitation was true always and everywhere in the whole universe. It was true in Seattle, where I had grown up with my family, and it was true in Cambridge, where I was struggling to find my way alone. Newton's was a mathematical universe, an infinite universe, a universe in which every time and every place was just like every other time and place.

Newton's world gave me strength. Every evening when classes were over, I would sit in the basement study of my dormitory and enter it. As I worked my physics problems, inertial balls rolled out of the infinite reaches of space past the place where I was sitting. I shrank myself to a point and observed them going steadily by, while the aged clock on the wall ticked off the seconds. My homesickness, my college, my being itself was ephemeral. There was something much larger and more steady at work in the world.

They would have laughed had I revealed my thoughts in the physics department, but Newton understood his mathematics and his physics as I did. He knew that all of our immediate knowledge of the world is contingent and costrained by our limitations; that we can experience only "relative" time and "relative" space. But Newton also understood that beyond all the time that we know, beyond all the space that we know, beyond all of everything that we know, was an absolute world—calm, clear, and undisturbed. "Absolute, true, and mathematical time, of itself and from its own nature, flows equably. . . . Absolute space, in its own nature, without realtion to anything external, remains always similar and immovable." At times Newton positively glowed with the peace of knowing things that were so true.

For me, Newton's mathematical space has long called to mind the words of one of Grandmama's favorite hymns. "Immortal, invisible, God only wise / In light inaccessible, hid from our eyes." The connection is not wholly idiosyncratic. Newton was acutely aware of the theological overtones of his views of time and space. He recognized that crucial adjectives—infinite, eternal, ever-present—applied equally to God and to his mathematical space and time. He reveled in this connection as much as he did in the mathematical power of the physics he constructed in absolute pure mathematical space. He described space as the "sensorium of God," almost God's brain itself. People cannot experience it directly ("in light inexpressible, hid from our eyes") but they are in the middle of it. Like space, God is always directly present to us all. He is mindful of His universe.

My Victorians would not have accepted the specifics of Newtonian theology, but many of them knew Newton's God. Their scientific work was suffused and sustained by the divine. I could just hear Grandmama's deep, well-modulated voice drawing her listeners along with the flowing sermonic prose of John Herschel, the most well-known spokesman for science in the early nineteenth century:

> There is something in the contemplation of general laws which power-fully persuades us to merge individual feeling, and to commit ourselves unreservedly to their disposal; while the observation of the calm, ener-getic regularity of nature, . . . tends, irresistibly, to tranquilize and re-assure the mind. . . And this it does . . . by filling us, as from an inward spring, with a sense of nobleness and power. [It forms] a link between ourselves and the best and noblest benefactors of our species, with whom we hold communion in thoughts and participate in discoveries which have . . . brought them nearer to their creator.

I am of a different world but as it often had in the past, my work with Victorian mathematicians served to tranquilize and reassure my mind on a very deep level. As I read and wrote in my office overlooking the semifrozen waters of the Charles River, I entered their space. In it, absolute, true, mathematical time flowed equably without reference to anything external.

At home I lived in an apparent, common space and time much less serene than Newton's mathematical one. There we were facing the uncertainties of seizure disorder. That is the new term for epilepsy. It was helpful to think of what Ned faced in this way; it was helpful to sep-arate our challenge from the stigma of centuries of fear. On the other hand, the change in term did not change the devastating combination of absolute demands with total unpredictability that the condition entails.

Rick and I got an inkling of this before we went skiing, when Dr. Lyman could not give a definite answer to virtually any of our questions about seizures. He did not know whether the Tegretol would block the seizures, whether it would blunt them, or whether Ned would have "breakthrough" seizures in any case. We would be aware of its failures, when or if they occurred: If Ned had a seizure, we would know that the Tegretol had not stopped it. If he did not, though, there was no way to know whether it was because the medication had blocked them or whether he just was not having seizures. The latter possibility could only be tested empirically by taking him off the Tegretol and seeing what happened then.

We were certainly not about to take Ned off Tegretol, so we moved on to the next set of questions, about how to know a seizure was coming and prepare for it. Here again the answers were elusive at best. Different people had different experiences that suggested they were in for a seizure and some had none. Ned described a visual experience as all he remembered of his seizure, and the more minor episodes I had related to Dr. Gasparian also involved some alteration of vision. This was in keeping with the location of the tumor, which was between the occipital and the temporal lobes of the brain. The temporal lobe is often the location of seizures and the occipital lobe is where sight is located. But there was very little time between the visual symptoms and the seizure—it seemed at most a matter of seconds. As a warning it was not helpful at all.

Dr. Lyman could offer nothing else by way of prognosticator, however.

"Could they be brought on by the fluorescent lights at school?"

"Maybe."

"Could it be the time of day? All the episodes he described were in the early afternoon."

"Maybe, but I doubt it."

"Could it be something he ate?"

"No. I wouldn't think so."

"Would being tired make them more likely?"

"Perhaps."

"So what do we do?"

"Well, for a while you just have to hope for the best and be prepared for the worst. In the next few months we will see how things develop. If Ned has more seizures, we can see whether there are any patterns we can identify in them."

Preparing for the worst was a bit daunting since a seizure of the magnitude Ned had experienced could be life-threatening in any number of situations. We got Ned a Medic Alert bracelet explaining the condition and giving appropriate phone numbers so that strangers could respond. We talked again to people at school. We talked to all of the neighbors. We hired additional after-school child-care. We talked to Ned about changing his behavior—no tree climbing, no bicycling, no rollerblading, no swimming, no baths without someone nearby.

Hoping for the best could be pretty difficult as well. It was not that we did not want it. Rather it was that we wanted it with such passion that we were in danger of crippling ourselves with denial, self-pity, or a combination of the two. Dr. Jennings's pre-Christmas decision not to operate was a great relief, and our skiing trip helped us to accept the wait. Still, the threat of seizures with all of their terrifying implications lay behind every day of our lives.

On the train that served as transitional time between the concretely immediate challenges of my private life and the quiet study of its public manifestation I wondered. De Morgan's distinction between the "moral" and the "mathematical" seemed almost physically located as I moved from Boston to Providence and back. I thought about the way he would look at Ned's situation. It required a bit of a stretch because Ned's situation did not fit directly into the mathematical model of probabilities De Morgan had constructed.

De Morgan had recognized that although we face uncertainty in many different situations, some are more uncertain than others. "It is more probable that rain will follow a fall of the barometer than a rise," he noted. This raised the question, "*how* much more probable?" De Morgan took as his challenge assigning precise numerical values to the various degrees of more or less; we can see the influence of his kind of program in the weather forcasters who tell us that there is a 30 percent chance of rain today.

Getting to this point required creating a model for the way we think about future events. De Morgan drew his from gambling. His favorite example was that of an urn filled with black and white balls. Making decisions in uncertain circumstances, he wrote, is like drawing balls from the urn in hopes of getting a black one. A rational person faced with betting in this situation will consider the proportion of black balls in the urn. If half of the balls are black, he or she can expect that blacks will be drawn half of the time. If two-thirds are black, he or she can expect black balls to be drawn two-thirds of the time. The thoughtful gambler will base any decisions he or she makes on this kind of probabilistic calculation. De Morgan thought that the truly rational decision maker would do the same. Given any situation with an unknown outcome, he or she would calculate the odds and decide accordingly.

From this vantage point, though, the challenge of Ned's seizures required a somewhat nonstandard approach. With De Morgan's urn, the assumption is that you know the ratio of black to white balls. What you don't know is the color of the ball that will be drawn in a particular instant. But Ned's seizures presented the problem in reverse. We did not know how often he might have seizures, we had no idea of the ratio of white to black balls in the urn. That is what we were trying to learn from experience, that is what I was trying to map as I recorded his seizure feelings in the little yellow notebook. Each seizure feeling constituted a black ball.

But, I realized as the train clattered along, I didn't know whether our urn contained just black or white balls or whether it housed a rainbow collection. I really had no clear idea of what constituted a black ball, what constituted a seizure. Did headaches count? What about vague feelings of malaise? Or did nothing count except a full-blown grand mal seizure? On the other hand, there was a question of what constituted a white ball; what was a nonseizure? a seizure-free week? day? schoolday? lunch hour? Questions crowded in from all sides, and on the Cambridge leg of the journey I defined, calculated, and scribbled ideas. But the closer I got to Providence, the more meaningless the whole exercise became.

"How was your day today, Ned?"

"Oh, fine. I didn't feel like playing outside so I made some cookies instead."

What did it mean that Ned didn't want to play outside? I didn't know so I let the issue drop. But every two or three weeks Ned reported "seizure feelings." These occurred with absolutely no rhyme or reason and persisted even though we raised the Tegretol levels slightly. Still none of the feelings was serious enough to interrupt his day. I noted the dates and his descriptions on the "Seizure" page of the little yellow notebook.

"Fuzzy vision." "Enhanced vision." The phrases were strikingly descriptive coming from my nine-year-old boy. They left no doubt that something uniquely powerful was happening. They captured the way I saw our lives as well, sometimes with startling clarity, sometimes with considerable confusion. As with the seizure feelings, however, moments of insight and moments of despair were not the norm. In my kitchen in the late afternoon the probabilities and certainties defined by all the urn exercises were absurd. Then and there the certainty was that Ned was fine, the kitchen was a mess, and dinner had to be brought together.

Decision

Dr. Jennings's pause gave us some time to make concrete plans for the upcoming trip to Germany. Brady, Rick, and I enrolled in German courses—Brady in first-year courses, Rick in second, and me in third. Brady never really engaged the problem; it's hard to believe a foreign language exists with no experience of it; Rick cheerfully moved through his weekly classes; I sat rather discombobulated in mine, having not thought of German as a spoken language since a college course more than twenty-five years before. In any case, we each spent an evening a week struggling with noun declensions and unfamiliar sentence constructions.

Day by day, the time passed. In January we celebrated Rick's forty-ninth birthday—roast chicken, wild rice, garlic bread, salad, and angel food cake. In February we celebrated Ned's tenth birthday—stir-fry chicken and vegetables, rice, chocolate cake, and chocolate-chip cookie-dough ice cream. Then came March, and the respite was over. We had to face Ned's tumor again.

"Neurosurgery. Dr. Jennings's office."

"Hello. My son, Edward Richards, has an appointment to see Dr. Jennings next Wednesday. Dr. Jennings asked that we get him a new set of MRI pictures, which we have done. I was just calling to check that you still have the set that we brought at Christmas so he can compare them at our appointment."

"Just a minute. . . . No, Mrs. Richards. We do not have anything here."

"But we left them with you right before Christmas."

"They are not here."

"Do you have any idea where they are?"

"Mrs. Richards, we do not have them here."

"Could I speak to Dr. Jennings? Maybe he knows where they are."

"They are not here, Mrs. Richards."

I was in tears when I called Janet, Dr. Lyman's secretary, for backup. "I do not know what the problem is," I confessed. "Maybe this is something that patients aren't supposed to ask. Perhaps you would have better luck getting them to focus on the problem of where Ned's pictures are."

Janet was as warm as the man for whom she worked. At one point Dr. Lyman explained to me that he and she were bound by a common philosophy, that the way you said things was as important as what you said in dealing with patients. It seems a simplistic way to summarize the woman who was such a mainstay to us through all of our medical woes. It was in the interaction with Dr. Jennings's secretaries that she first proved her mettle.

"Don't worry, Mrs. Richards," the ever-cheerful and efficient woman said. "I'll call."

She did, but reached the same dead end in her attempts to communicate with the Boston women that I had. Undaunted, she went on to call the office where the pictures had been taken originally to see whether copies could be made. It was then that she found that the pictures were already there in Ned's file. Though his secretaries treated the practice as if it were classified information, Dr. Jennings routinely returned MRIs to their place of origin. On the way to our appointment, I picked them up from the radiologist's office.

A cluster of tense family groups sat miserably in the crowded hall outside of Dr. Jennings's door. Children, toddlers, and teenagers vied for the outdated magazines while their parents tried to avoid each other's eyes. Some of the children looked as fine as Ned, others had scars on their shaved heads, others had neurological problems that were expressed in twitches or other noticeable behavior. Into Dr. Jennings's office they went and then emerged. Some left, silent and grim; some proceeded to the secretaries' lair to make surgical appointments; one grinned at her toddler and said, "Did you hear that, Suzy? You do not have to see another surgeon for a whole year!" Rick, Ned, and I feigned interest in our cast-off reading material and waited.

"Edward Richards."

Dr. Jennings was a very precise, clean-shaven man, somewhere between fifty-five and sixty. His office was crowded with things—books, files, papers, pictures, inspirational sayings . . . One saying hung high above his bookcases on the wall facing his desk; as he faced a patient, Dr. Jennings could always look up to see "Lord, Let me be an instrument of thy peace." Dr. Jennings's manner was as precise as his appearance—and equally at odds with his physical environment. As he questioned us, seated behind his relatively clear desk, a host of carefully learned lessons in seminars called things like "Sensitive Patient Interaction" clicked away behind his disciplined eyes.

He took Ned and the two sets of MRIs into an adjoining room. We remained seated in the main office while through the open door we could see Ned staring into lights, walking straight lines, and kicking when hammered. Then, Dr. Jennings sent Ned back and we all watched through the open door while the doctor studied the pictures. After about two minutes he returned to his place behind the desk.

"Well," he said. "It could be several things. It could be . . ."

I prepared to take notes in my little yellow notebook. Dr. Jennings looked at me questioningly.

"I just forget things," I explained. "It helps to write them down."

"Yes, but I'm not sure about what I am saying. I cannot really identify what this is from the pictures."

"I know." I tried to reassure him. "I'll write on the page 'Dr. Jennings thinks it *might be* . . .'"

Mollified he began again. "It is peculiar," he said. "It is very bright—too bright to be a meningioma." The best and most benign hope offered by Dr. Harlow was gone. "It looks like some kind of benign lesion," he went on. "Maybe some kind of hamartoma, PXA, a glioma . . ." The terms were becoming more familiar. I clung to "benign" as I carefully wrote them down.

"Has it grown?"

"I don't know. Maybe a little."

"Then we don't have to operate?"

"Well, we could operate or we could wait and see what happens. We could monitor it every six months for a while."

Rick and I waited, breathlessly hopeful.

"I think we should do a CAT scan," he said. "It may seem a technological step backward, but sometimes we see things there we can't on an MRI. It is more familiar."

He rose. We shook hands. All the eyes in the hall turned toward us as we walked out. I do not know what they read on our faces but we were very happy. It had not grown, at least not perceptibly; certainly that meant it could not be terribly malignant. We were not making a surgical appointment. Ned seemed to have at least one foot out of the woods.

It took about two weeks to get the computerized axial tomography, or CAT, scan. The process was quiet and for this reason less daunting than the MRI. As soon as I had them, I dropped the pictures off in Dr. Jennings's office.

On Thursdays Rick had Ned's Cub Scout meeting in the house. They were a rowdy bunch, and things worked better when I wasn't there. Whenever I could I worked late on Thursdays.

Rick was subdued when he picked me up at the night train. He told me about the Cub Scout craft project. I commiserated about the difficulties of maintaining constructive calm with a group of nine-year-old boys.

"Oh!" It came almost as an afterthought. "Dr. Jennings called. He wants to operate on Ned."

"What?! Why didn't you say so before? What is the problem? What happened? What was wrong with the CAT scan he didn't know before?" Questions exploded out of me.

"I don't know, Joan," Rick said wearily. "He called in the middle of the meeting and the kids were acting up. Besides I don't think of all your questions when I talk to him. You're the one who writes it all down. I can't think at all about this. He's going to call you tomorrow."

Through the hours, minutes, seconds, of that Friday I polished silver, sorted spices, and cleaned kitchen cabinets, all the while thinking of De Morgan and his urns of colored balls. While I kept waiting for the phone to ring, my thoughts turned again and again to a single example on a single page of his *Theory of Probabilities*. In that passage—just one example among the endless mathematical arguments and calculations that pack his ninety-seven folio pages—De Morgan considers the situation of a man who is sitting before an urn filled with black and white balls. If a black ball is drawn, he will die. For this man there would be an infinite difference between an urn with no black balls and an urn that contains only one. De Morgan used his plight as an example of "moral probability," an example to show that if you have a deep personal stake in a situation, "mathematical probabilities" do not make sense.

As I cut new shelf paper for the kitchen cabinets, I recognized that Rick and I were living the situation of De Morgan's condemned person, facing the devastation of even a single black ball. But, it was crucial to Ned's health, not to say life, that we make a right decision. Surely, we could remove ourselves enough from our emotional commitments to act rationally. Surely we could control ourselves enough to see the truth that was greater than our fear. When the phone rang at about three-thirty I was carefully washing the tops of each of my spice bottles.

"Hello, Mrs. Richards? This is Dr. Jennings. I have looked at the MRIs and the CAT scans for your son, Edward. As I told your husband, I think we should operate."

"Why?"

"The lesion is small but it is right on the Labe vein. If it were to grow, it could become dangerous and much more difficult to remove."

"OK. But what are the counterindications to the operation?"

"Well, the worst that could happen would be damage to the Labe vein. That might mean loss of communication centers."

"What do you mean?"

"He would have trouble processing speech—knowing the meaning of what was said to him, being able to communicate his ideas. But this will not happen, Mrs. Richards: I will not cut the Labe vein."

"You mean he will not be able to understand or communicate but will in all other ways be normal? He'll be an active vegetable?"

"Mrs. Richards. This will not happen. I have to tell you what are the worst possibilities. That does not mean they will happen."

"OK. Are there other possibilities?"

"If there is a massive hemorrhage, he might suffer a field-cut."

"What does that mean?"

"It means that he would lose some portion of his vision. If you think of what you see as a circular field, some portion of it would be occluded—anywhere from a small wedge to the whole half, depending on how massive the hemorrhage. This is harder to predict, but I am quite sure there will not be a massive hemorrhage. He may lose some sight on the left side, but not the whole hemisphere."

"He would lose vision on the left side?"

"Yes. The sides of the brain control different sides of the body. Since the lesion is on the right, it would affect the left side of his vision."

I was startled. "On the *right*? It is on the *left*."

"Mrs. Richards, I have looked at the pictures. It is on the *right* side of the brain."

"But everyone else said the *left*."

"Mrs. Richards." His voice was firm, clipped, and irritated. I was going to get nowhere by arguing the point, so I moved to my next question.

"If we decided to operate, how soon would it be?"

"It takes six to eight weeks to schedule an operation of this kind."

"My brother is a radiologist," I said. "He is concerned about his nephew and would like to look at the pictures. Could I send them to him in the interim? I could certainly have them back in six weeks."

"Of course. Let me get them." I could hear Dr. Jennings shuffling through papers in the background.

"Mrs. Richards?"

"Yes."

"I made a mistake. The lesion is on the *left* side of the brain."

"Yes," I said, relieved. "Does that change the decision to operate?"

"I do not want to talk about it now. I will call you back."

"Because the left side is the more important side for a right-handed person, would that affect the advice you've given so far?"

"Mrs. Richards, I have to reconsider the situation. I will not answer any more questions until I have done that."

He hung up.

An hour later the phone rang again.

"Mrs. Richards, I took Edward's pictures to our head of radiology, Dr. Simons. We looked at them very carefully together. The lesion is on the left side of the brain. It was something else that I saw on the right side of the brain but we agreed that it is not a significant object. I then took them to Dr. Rogers, one of my neurosurgical colleagues. We agreed that because of its location on the Labe vein it is advisable to operate before it gets any larger. So my advice is the same as it was before."

"Are the risks any different because it is the left rather than the right?"

"No. The only difference is that if there were a field cut it would be on the right instead of the left of his field of vision. But I do not think there will be a field cut, Mrs. Richards."

"OK."

"Shall I tell Meghan to schedule the operation?"

"No, Dr. Jennings. I have to talk the situation over with my husband and Dr. Lyman."

"All right, Mrs. Richards. I can understand that. But I want to be perfectly clear about my opinion. It is important that this lesion be removed soon. If it were to grow, it could become inoperable."

"Thank you, Dr. Jennings. I understand your position."

I hung up overwhelmed. I did not know how to think about the operation; I knew even less about how to respond to Dr. Jennings's mistake. It was so shocking, so egregious, and yet so human. I did not dare tell anyone but Rick about it. He did not know how to respond either and simply put it aside. I lay wide-eyed in the night. It was almost two weeks before we could get an appointment with Dr. Lyman to discuss our choices. He scheduled us in the evening so that we could have as much time as we needed to examine the issue from all sides.

The doctor did not schedule Ned's next major seizure, but it occurred on the same day as our appointment. Ned had wakened that

Wednesday morning in early April vaguely out of sorts and unwilling to go to school. As luck would have it I had no specific conflicting appointments, and so, softened by my knowledge of the major issues he was facing, I arranged to work at home. We spent a quiet morning; I remember being warmed by his laughing aloud at some book he was reading as I brought accounts up to date in the next room. For lunch we had chicken soup with rice, a favorite since the days when we read Maurice Sendak together—"Eating once, eating twice, eating chicken soup with rice." Ned was not particularly hungry but pecked at his bowl of soup while I ate mine. Suddenly he hurled himself out of his chair in great distress. "It's happening! It's happening! I can't stop it, Mom! I can't stop it! It's happening!" he cried as he lurched toward the stove.

Mind whirling, I caught Ned from behind so he would not hit his head in a fall. He continued to cry while I decided to risk taking him into his bedroom. It seemed less hard and cold than the kitchen floor. It was not far and I succeeded in maneuvering Ned onto his bed. I sat on the side ready to prevent him from throwing himself out of it, were major convulsions to start. They did not. He lay terrified and staring, losing his vision but not his hearing. I talked to him.

"It's OK, Ned. You may go away for a while but I am not going anywhere. I am right here and I am not going anywhere. I will be here even if you don't know it for a little while. I am right here. I am not going anywhere."

"But I can't see! It's all green! I can't see my room!"

"It's OK, Ned. Soon you will see again. The room is still here. And I am right here. I am not going away. I am right here."

After about five minutes Ned's vision began to return. He was still frightened and agitated, but I felt I could risk a quick call to the doctor.

"Dr. Lyman's office."

"Hello, this is Joan Richards, Ned's mother. He is having another seizure."

"I'm going to transfer you to a nurse, Mrs. Richards."

The transfer was immediate. I repeated my situation to the listening nurse.

"You mean a full-scale seizure, Mrs. Richards?"

"Well, he has not lost consciousness nor did he have convulsions, but something major has happened."

"OK, you'd better bring him in."

"Bring him in? But he is limp and exhausted. I can't bring him in like this!"

"Does he need an ambulance?"

"No, I guess not."

"OK. Bring him in. Dr. Lyman has appointments this afternoon, but one of the other doctors will see him."

In the background I heard Janet's cheerful, strong voice. "Fiddlesticks! Of course Dr. Lyman will see him. We can swap the schedules."

I put down the back seat of our station wagon and lined it with blankets and a pillow. Then I maneuvered Ned and Racky, his beloved stuffed raccoon, into it. He lay still and whimpered as we drove to the doctor's office. A more sensible person than I spotted us staggering across the parking lot and raced up with a wheelchair. Ned slumped in it, Racky at his side, and I wheeled him to Dr. Lyman's office. Janet was standing at the door ready to whisk us past the concerned denizens of the waiting room to Dr. Lyman. Ned was quickly transferred to an examining table. Dr. Lyman held the wastebasket and I held Ned's head as he vomited.

The afternoon unfolded with more of the same. I drove and wheeled the periodically vomiting Ned from specialist to specialist, who checked him from top to bottom and found no new developments. There was no hemorrhage, the tumor had not changed, there was no evidence of neurological damage. At about five o'clock, just as the barrage of tests was winding down, Ned felt better. He offered to race me down the corridor of the radiologist's office—me on foot, he with Racky in the chair.

For Ned the seizure may have been over, but for his parents, and his doctors, it was not. This incident demonstrated to Rick and me that the situation could not just be allowed to lie. Even on Tegretol, Ned was liable to have serious seizures and they were no picnic. In fact, in some ways the milder, Tegretol-muted seizure was worse than the full-scale one. That Ned did not lose consciousness might have been a comfort to witnesses, but it was not necessarily so for him. Rather than emerging totally unscathed except for an hour sliced from his time, he carried away the memory of an experience terrifying in the extreme.

That evening, when we returned for our appointment with Dr. Lyman, it was clear to us all that the surgery, which before seemed almost too awful to contemplate, might be worth it. But it was very hard to know how to make a decision of this magnitude. I tried framing the situation with probabilities.

"Is there any way to know what the risks are in this kind of situation? Are there any statistics on the incidence of neurological damage with this kind of surgery? Or is each case so unique that such statistics don't say anything?"

Dr. Lyman's answer shattered De Morgan's urn, and with it all thought of rational calculation. "I don't know whether there are such statistics, but even if there were, I think a surgeon would say that they are irrelevant. Any good, self-confident surgeon would say, 'That may be the case for surgeons in general but not for me.' I've referred you to Dr. Jennings because of his record."

I took a deep breath, hardly daring to raise the question of Dr. Jennings's mistake. All of the people we had consulted pointed to him as Ned's best hope. We needed his skills so much, it was terrifying. But he had made such a frighteningly significant error that I could not just ignore it as we discussed our options with Dr. Lyman.

"Dr. Lyman? If we had this operation, is Dr. Jennings the best person to do it?"

Dr. Lyman's open visage became alert and studiedly receptive. "Why do you ask?" he wondered. I told him about my conversations with Dr. Jennings. When I finished, he admitted that he already knew what had happened.

"Dr. Jennings called me after he talked to you. He said he had made a mistake about the location of the lesion. He made it clear that he thinks it is important that this operation be done soon. If you do not want him to do it, he can recommend people in New York, in Chicago, in Toronto, who can do it."

Rick and I looked at each other long and hard. New York? Chicago? Toronto? An unknown surgeon in a strange town?

"You may go wherever you want. But you should know that Dr. Jennings's error was one on the level of patient interaction. The time that he really studies the pictures is with the whole operating team, in the hour before the surgery. It is as a surgeon that he is so well thought of."

Rick and I continued to try to ask intelligent questions, but it was a human conversation, devoid of calculated rationality. We had to make a decision based on our trust in Dr. Lyman and, through him, Dr. Jennings. After about fifteen additional minutes we committed our son to the great unknown of neurosurgery.

Surgery

"I would like to make a surgical appointment with Dr. Jennings for my son, Edward Richards."

"Oh, yes, Mrs. Richards. I will set that up as soon as I can and get back to you about it."

"Thank you."

"Hello, Mrs. Richards. I have scheduled surgery for Edward on Tuesday, May 30. You will have to bring him up for a preoperative checkup the week before."

"Can we have an appointment with Dr. Jennings before that?"

"Did Dr. Jennings say he wanted to see you, Mrs. Richards?"

"Yes. He said he wanted to see us before the operation."

"OK, Mrs. Richards. He can see you in three weeks, April 29 at eleven-fifteen."

"Hello, Mrs. Richards. This is Meghan from Dr. Jennings's office. Dr. Jennings has an emergency and he cannot see you today at eleven-fifteen."

"Oh! Well . . . can we reschedule?"

"You want to reschedule?"

"Yes. Dr. Jennings said he would talk to us before our son's operation."

"OK. Let's see. . . . He can see you in eight weeks, on June 8 at twelve-fifteen."

"But that is *after* the operation!"

"Oh. You're right. I'll squeeze you in on Thursday, May 26 at four."

I stayed calm with Dr. Jennings's brusquely changeable secretaries but inside, with all of my being, I feared for Ned.

The world turned grim. One morning in my Cambridge office I idly allowed myself to be distracted by a chugging helicopter in its flight over the Charles River. Then, without reason, it sputtered, stopped, and crashed onto the shore in front of me. Newton's laws held without exception; the vehicle traced a perfect parabolic curve in its descent but I found no beauty in it. I went home early to avoid watching the grisly process of clearing up the debris and the dead.

Later in the spring I was thrilled by a hawk who sat on the limb of a tree outside my window. I sat still and watched, entranced by his noble strength. He shifted on the branch and stared back. Then he looked down disdainfully and shifted again. His claws were large enough to obliterate my view of all but the tail of a small squirrel whose twitching was disturbing him. I fled to the library as the bird meditatively dismembered and ate the squirrel child.

I kept trying to work. One afternoon, as I was consulting De Morgan's wife's *Memoir*, I was startled by a rare personal note: "I did not, for my part, endeavour to influence him in this matter. Indeed, at this time my whole thoughts were filled most painfully by the illness of our eldest child, whose danger was not at first realized by her father."

Curious, I read beyond the paragraph surrounding the collegiate incident, to see whether Sophia's concerns about their child's health were mentioned further. The next paragraph devastated me. "The end of this year was the beginning of a long period of sorrow and suffering to us. Our eldest dear child, Alice, who had caught cold after a severe attack of measles, died before Christmas. I had feared the termination of the great weakness and delicacy which I had vainly tried to prevent. Her father did not realise the degree of illness till the end was near and the blow fell heavily upon him. . . . He always dwelt on the belief that those whom God loves are the early taken, but after we lost Alice his cheerfulness diminished, and I do not think he ever laughed so heartily, or was heard whistling and singing merry snatches of songs as he used to do when all our children were with us. I cannot write of these events."

Sophia could barely write of them; I could barely read of them. I spent the rest of my afternoon piecing together seven children from scattered references in the *Memoir*. Three of them predeceased their father. All of his rationality, wit, and intelligence could do nothing to save them.

In the night I lay awake . . . twelve, twelve-thirty, one. I got up and went to the kitchen where the light would bother no one. Grandmama's cherub gazed sympathetically from his sunburst frame as I opened the calculus text I kept stashed among the cookbooks. I found a problem to solve:

1. Find dz/dt for $z = x^2 - 2xy + y^2$, $x = (t + 1)^2$, $y = (t - 1)^2$

"Well, this needs the chain rule: $dz/dt = \partial z/\partial x\, dx/dt + \partial z/\partial y\, dy/dt$. OK, dx/dt is just $2(t + 1)$ and dy/dt is $2(t - 1)$. Now $\partial z/\partial x$ would be $2x - 2y$ and . . ."

Rick came in and joined me at the table. "It's hard to sleep without you."

I warmed milk with maple syrup; we sipped quietly together. "Six o'clock is only three hours away. Let's give it another try."

I wrote to the *Wissenschaftskolleg*, warning that we simply might not be able to come. Ned's reports of "fuzzy vision" and "enhanced vision" increased, as did reports of severe headaches. The latter were a bit hard to classify since he claimed to have some kind of a headache virtually all the time. His activity level did not decrease, however: he went faithfully to school and we exorcised demons with homework projects; a relief map of the state of Oregon, a trip to the Boston Museum of Fine Arts for a report on the Egyptians.

On the weekends Ned worked in his garden. When he was three he had talked to flowers so volubly that Rick had cut a rectangle out of the middle of our small urban backyard to be Ned's own. Every year Ned cheered a rugged group of vegetables to maturity in the shadow of the neighbor's maple tree.

At ten Ned was not as conversational with the vegetables as he had been at four or five. But the process of choosing the new cast of characters was an important part of every spring. "We got eggplant this year, Mom! And red peppers!" Digging in the compost, laying out the rows, planting different plants at different times kept Ned and Rick busy and dirty, weekend after weekend. "We put in the lettuce, Mom, but it's too cold for the tomatoes. We'll have to leave them in the window for a while."

Brady began rowing with his equally tall friend, Matt. The rest of us threw ourselves into Little League. At ten, Ned's league allowed the children to pitch to one another for the first time and he, like all of the other members of the team, longed to be a pitcher. The coach's child, an athletic girl named Christine, was an excellent pitcher—the starter. Backup positions were much contested, though, and Ned practiced with Rick in hopes of qualifying. Alas, though possessed of a strong arm and a good aim, Ned also has a fierce and volatile temper. The first time the coach put Ned on the mound he walked two runners on balls and then stalked off the mound in a black rage. This did not prove to be an effective strategy for persuading the coach that Ned was valuable as a pitcher. Thereafter Ned was catcher to Christine's pitching: after her three-inning limit these two would be put together to pasture in left field. They became fast friends, rejoicing together over triumphs, commiserating over irritations that focused on Christine's occasional bad innings and on Ned's frustrated desire to be given a chance on the mound. He continued to practice with Rick, and game after game he hoped to pitch, but the coach never forgave his initial loss of composure.

We had not made a big issue about Ned's seizures or his impending surgery at Little League; it seemed a good place to have things completely normal. One of us was always there in case there was a problem, but for most of the season we said nothing. However, the scheduled surgery did mean that he would miss the two final games of the season. In the last week I told this to the coach; it seemed at that time a necessary piece of information so the man could make adjustments to the lineup. He duly made a note of it, but did not seem otherwise interested in whatever issues might be facing this member of his team.

Ned was acutely aware of his last game, however, and desperate to be allowed to pitch once more. He showed up eager to try and presented his case to the coach. The man brushed him off brusquely and for the first inning Ned donned the catcher's uniform. At the second inning he tried again to get some time on the mound—again he was dismissed. The third inning he again was catcher. With the fourth inning came a mandatory pitching change and Ned flung himself into the argument that he be allowed to pitch. The coach chose another player and sent Ned and Christine into the field. Ned stamped and pouted and picked dandelions. He fielded a ball, one of his teammates fumbled it, and Ned yelled at him. He threw his glove on the field in a rage, forcing Christine to field a ball in his territory. He yelled at her for taking "his" ball.

At this point a Little League official decided Ned needed to be brought into line. At the change of inning he called Ned over and began to dress him down. I did not know what my role was in the male world of baseball, so I decided to let things take their course. Ned certainly was not behaving well and the man might be able to reach him. When the man ran out of breath, Ned turned on him.

"How can you tell me how to behave?" he yelled. "You have never been in a situation like mine! You have never even had a seizure! Well, I have, and they are terrible! You have never had a brain tumor either! Well, I have, and it is very scary! You have never had to have neurosurgery either: no one has ever said they were going to cut your skull open! Well that's what Dr. Jennings is going to do to me on Tuesday! And you won't even let me pitch! I just wanted to pitch one time before they operated on me and you won't even let me try. Just because I made a mistake once you will not ever let me try again! Well I hate you and I hate this game and I am leaving!"

The official was staggered, the coach was staggered, and I was staggered. Ned turned on his heel and climbed into the car. There was little else to say.

As well as marking the termination of his baseball season, Ned's outburst marked a turning point for the family. His cheerful resilience had long protected all of us from what was about to happen to him, but now Rick could not pun and I could not laugh. Brady emerged from his room. We all went for Ned's preoperative visit to the hospital and his final appointment with Dr. Jennings.

"Dr. Jennings is still in the operating room. He will not be able to see you today."

"But he said he would see us before the operation!"

"Mrs. Richards, Dr. Jennings is a very busy man. He operates on children with brain tumors. It is very important work. He does not have time to see you."

"Surgical call."

"Hello, this is Dr. Richards. I would like to speak to Dr. Jennings. I can be reached at 407-555-1469."

"Hello, this is Dr. Jennings. May I please speak to Dr. Richards?"

"Hello Dr. Jennings. This is Dr. Richards. I am the mother of Edward Richards. You are going to operate on my son on Tuesday and you said we would see you before the operation. You could not keep your appointment today and your secretaries could not find another time for us to meet."

"Mrs. Richards! You have no right to page me in this way. You can make your appointments with me through my secretaries."

"But sir, they said you had no time to see us. You said you wanted to see us before the surgery and it is very important to me that I see you before the operation. I will not bring my son in on Tuesday unless I've seen you."

"OK, Mrs. Richards. Of course I will see you. Let's see. I'm leaving town at nine-thirty tomorrow morning and will not be back until Monday night."

"I can meet you in the airport, if you like."

"Don't be silly. I will see you in the hospital tomorrow morning at seven-thirty."

"Thank you, Dr. Jennings."

"You could have arranged this through my secretaries."

"Thank you, Dr. Jennings."

As Rick and I waited in Dr. Jennings's hall, I overheard the doctor explaining our early-morning presence to his colleagues: "She said she was a doctor but she was really a mother."

Our appointment was a strained five minutes long. Rick had come only out of loyalty to me, and had nothing to say. I didn't have much to say either, but I hadn't come to talk anyway. What I needed was to see once more the person to whom I was entrusting Ned's life. As Dr. Jennings again scolded me for reaching him and curtly answered a short list of manufactured questions, I looked at his hands.

Memorial Day weekend stretched an interminably long three days before us: "I'm taking the dog for a walk," "This afternoon we can go to a movie!" "My mother comes tomorrow." "Can we can go to another movie?" "I'm going to work in the garden." "Let's go for a walk." "I'm going to take a nap." "Leave me alone!" "Is it only ten-thirty? We can't have lunch yet!" "I'm going to the bookstore to find a book." Minute by minute, time crept by.

Tuesday morning at five o'clock we could finally do something. Ned was excited and eagerly climbed into the car holding his allowance of two carefully selected stuffed animals. Brady and my mother waved us away from the front porch. Rick drove the car resolutely to Boston.

We were right on time for our six o'clock appointment with the pre-operative department. Five days before, they had run a whole series of tests. This morning there was little to be done but dress Ned in a gown and put matching bands on him and his animals. We then marched down various corridors to a room and a bed, where Ned waited with a couple of other children for the doctors. At about seven o'clock the anesthesiologist arrived to give him a sedative. Dr. Jennings showed up about fifteen minutes later and asked whether we had any further questions. Then they wheeled our by-now-sleeping Ned away.

Rick and I faced the estimated five hours until the operation would be over in a large, unmistakably institutional waiting room with about twenty disparate configurations of waiting family groups. The nurse who presided over us all relayed reports she received every hour and a half from each operation in progress. At nine o'clock she told Rick and me that the incision had been made fifteen minutes before. I tried not to think of the process involved in making an incision for brain surgery. At ten-thirty she told us that Dr. Jennings was working under a microscope and all seemed to be going well. I went for a walk and sat in a hospital chapel to calm my nerves. I was just about to ask for the next informational fix, as twelve o'clock moved toward twelve-fifteen, when Dr. Jennings appeared, as calm and precise as ever in his green surgical scrubs. He took us into a small cubicle where he told us that the operation had gone as well as it possibly could have. There was very little bleeding and he thought he had gotten the entire tumor out.

"There might be a few cells left, close to the Labe vein. I did not want to scrape it down too hard," he clarified, "but I don't think so. The pathologist said it seemed to be a pilocytic astrocytoma; I would have said PXA—it looked yellow to me—but we can wait for the final report. In either case, it is benign and I think I got it out."

The doctor smiled and shook our hands. He then showed Rick and me how to get to the intensive-care unit and was gone.

The surgeon was content, but to the parental eye, a child in the intensive-care unit is a sobering sight. Ned lay half-asleep and very pale in a large room, broken into individual areas by banks of monitoring devices. His bed made an angle with that of another child who had had a tracheotomy. A nurse sat at the apex of the angle formed by the two children's feet. Her full-time job was to watch the two of them. Ned had an intravenous line in each arm, an additional arterial line in the left one. His naked chest was studded with metallic stickers that were hooked to machines measuring heart rate, breathing rate, and other vital signs. His face was surrounded by the same shock of hair with which we had delivered him to Dr. Jennings. But when he turned his head on the pillow there was a startling shaved line from the top of his head into the nape of his neck that was covered with a pressure bandage. The incision, we later ascertained, ran from a point just to the left of his cowlick down the back of his head and about an inch into his neck. It was a good six inches long, closed with twenty extraordinarily neat stitches.

The twenty-four hours in intensive care remained uneventful for Ned. Rick and I spent the night in the room the hospital provided for people like us: a large space divided by curtains into four cubicles. Each cubicle had some strange configuration of cots and linens for two; early to bed, Rick and I picked the one in which the beds seemed the least broken, pulled the curtain around us, and tried to sleep. As is his wont,

Rick succeeded better than I. I woke at about midnight to his familiar gentle snores and the appalled comment from someone in another cubicle: "Is he going to go on like that all night?" I poked him; he turned over and was still. I padded out to check on Ned who was also still, and came back to try to sleep again.

The next morning a neurologist, Dr. Pencraft, appeared at Ned's bedside to put him through an extensive series of tests to check for neurological damage. After about fifteen minutes of gentle banter, games, and questions, the doctor pronounced Ned completely normal. He warned us that in the next week or two Ned might develop neurological symptoms because of swelling, but assured us that Ned would eventually return to the baseline just established. That baseline was absolutely perfect: our relief was palpable.

At noon, a scant twenty-four hours after his operation, Ned was transferred from intensive care to "Ten South," the neurosurgical ward. Here he shared a room with a toddler; he had the window bed that overlooked a massive parking lot construction project. By this time he was alert for considerable periods; immediately upon arrival he turned on his TV only to find that the hospital channel featured the minutia of the same construction project. Disappointed, he alternately read and snoozed for the afternoon. My mother and Brady showed up to marvel at how well he seemed. Brady was soon engrossed in a video; Ned dozed on and off by his side. Rick, my mother, and I escaped the hospital for an hour and a cup of coffee.

Escape was definitely in order. Ten South was one of the most awful places I've ever been. Ned's tiny roommate was there for a series of tests to find out whether her seizures were the result of a terminal genetic disease. The child's mother, who was pregnant, was herself being tested to see whether her unborn child was afflicted as well. Because of the total lack of privacy imposed by a room where beds are divided only by a curtain, we were forced to listen to the whole dreadful tale as it unfolded.

At one point a doctor entered the room. "Hello, I'm Dr. Murdoch. I'm a geneticist working on your daughter's case. I need to ask you a few questions about your pregnancy."

The mother exploded. "I have already told six people about my pregnancy in the past twenty-four hours! Can't you ask one of them?"

"No," the man replied gently. "We all have to take our own histories. That way if one of us makes a mistake or leaves something out, the error won't be preserved and passed on."

"OK, I understand," the woman said bravely, and launched again into the painful tale she had told so many times before.

When her husband returned, she burst into tears behind the curtain. "How could I have been so rude and impatient?" she sobbed. "What must the doctors think of me?"

I bit my lip and left the room, but the view from the hall was not much better. Most children were in bed, hooked up to machines of all descriptions. Some of those who were ambulatory sported veritable roadmaps of scars on their shaved heads. Others seemed fine, but you knew they could not be; no one even remotely healthy would spend time on Ten South.

The next morning, Ned was unhooked from his various lines and encouraged to walk a bit. His first foray was a wobbly trip to the end of the corridor; by noon he ventured to the cafeteria for lunch; by late afternoon he teetered between Rick and me around a sweet garden surrounded on all sides by towering hospital buildings. At six in the evening he was given a postoperative MRI. At about seven-thirty Dr. Jennings came into the room.

"Hello, Edward, how are you doing?"

"Fine."

"Nice balloons you have. Have you been walking around?"

"Yes, we went around the garden and looked at the statues."

"Good! Did you eat while you were there?"

"Yes, Dad got me a yogurt."

"How about the TV? Have you been watching it?"

"Yes, but the hospital programs are stupid. They keep showing pictures of the parking lot."

"Oh, well! Do you have something else to do? Have you been reading your books?"

"Yes, but they make me tired."

"Of course. But then you can go to sleep."

"Yup!"

"Can you do something for me? Look right at me, into my eyes. . . . Right. Now tell me. Is the door to the room open or closed? . . . Good. How about the door to the bathroom? . . . Good. Your peripheral vision—that's how well you see on the sides—is perfect."

Dr. Jennings turned to Rick and me.

"I spoke to Dr. Pencraft, the neurologist who checked Edward yesterday morning and he finds no neurological problems. I also see no problems. And the MRI shows what I had hoped—there is no sign of tumor cells."

"Thank God! . . . Oh Good! . . . Thank you, sir! . . . How much longer will he be staying here?"

"Well, he can go home now, if you like."

"You mean right now? You can check him out at seven-thirty in the evening?"

"Well, I was thinking in terms of tomorrow morning, but if you want to take him home now you could. It would be some kind of record to send a child home after only three days and two nights, but there is no reason he must be here."

"Thank you, Dr. Jennings. We will leave now."

"Fine. The paperwork will take about an hour. The nurses will give you the medicines and explain the steroid taper. In ten days someone should take out his stitches. And I would like to see him in four weeks."

"Thank you, Dr. Jennings."

Ned's recovery continued to be incredibly rapid. The unexpected blessing of brain surgery is that there are few muscles on the skull and no nerves reporting the brain's feeling, so the incision was virtually painless. On Saturday, four days after the operation, Rick prepared to take Ned for a haircut. Brady went too. "If my brother is going to be a skinhead, so will I!" he vowed, and he made the ultimate sacrifice. Ned slept exhaustedly after the outing. Brady hoarded the bathroom mirror as he worked up the courage to expose his newly bald state to his friends.

In less than two weeks Dr. Lyman removed Ned's stitches and Ned proudly showed off his startling scar in symbolic half days at school. His seizures vanished with the tumor and he did not show any signs of neurological damage. Dr. Jennings canceled our postoperative appointment but left word with his secretary that Ned could go to summer camp. The only restrictions were that he not engage in contact sports and not do high dives. It was very hard for us to let him go, but at the same time we could see that it was important that we treat Ned as normally as possible. Rick and I resolutely drove the three hours to New Hampshire and dropped our happy Ned off.

My mother flew home to the West Coast where Brady joined her as soon as school was finished. Rick went back to his work. I wrote to the *Wissenschaftskolleg* saying that we would be coming after all, and went back to my commuting life.

The Alice in Me

It was an odd limbo time. Had nothing at all happened?

I struggled to make sense of the medical relationships that had drawn in our very souls and then let us go without a backward glance. I heard Grandmama's clear, deep voice. "Manners maketh man," she said. I sent notes with flowers and fruit to Janet and Dr. Lyman.

Dr. Jennings posed a more difficult problem, though. Thank-you notes should be honest. I struggled to find the right letter for him.

June 5, 1995

Dear Dr. Jennings,

Home after the surgery you performed on Ned, I join the host of parents who thank you from the bottom of their hearts for a job well done. He seems well beyond our wildest hopes and we could not be more grateful.

This letter does not stop there, however. I remain troubled by the evening of May 25, when you cancelled our appointment because of an emergency, and I reached you through your beeper. You scolded me for crashing through your defenses to speak to you personally instead of relying on your secretaries. I apologize to both you and them if I was out of line in response to an inconvenience that was legitimate and beyond any of our control.

At the same time, I realize that my response was conditioned by my earlier experiences dealing with your office. I believe that there is a problem in the way you and your secretaries deal with your patients that you should all address. The issues are in some important way structural: there is a mismatch of concern between a busy doctor and an anxious parent, and your office stands on the line between the two. Still, it is a central part of your job to negotiate the boundary as well as possible. Your patients are by definition new to it and should not have to add dealing with your office to their concerns.

In my experience there are a number of problems with your current set-up which you and your secretaries could and should address. All are important to your patients, and none would be terribly difficult to remedy, . . .

The letter went on for two full pages. I tried to be balanced, helpful, clear.

"What!" my friends said. "No, Joan! You can't send that! You may have to work with him for years! What if he gets angry with you? What if he refuses to work with you any more? You need him! There is no one else!"

I hated being so absolutely dependent on someone so autocratic, but I knew they were right. I have never been so terrified of another human being as I was of Dr. Jennings. I had pushed him hard before the operation, but then I was *in extremis*; now I was not. Ned needed me to insure that he continued to receive the best possible care, not to tell Dr. Jennings how to behave. I did not dare to threaten our relationship in any way. I waited for time to bring perspective on our interactions.

In my office I needed perspective as well. I had two papers to finish, the pathetic output of a whole year's work. My year's sabbatical seemed to have confirmed my colleagues' judgment that I was not worth promoting. Even now, with Ned apparently fine, I found that I could not settle down to work on my book. I could manage specific tasks, like rewriting a final paragraph or organizing a bibliography, but more general interest in my mathematicians could not compete with the noises in my head that were reviewing the past, clinging to the precarious present, and anticipating the unknown future.

After some painful attempts to hold my nose to the grindstone, I gave up. It was only a scant two months until the boys and I were moving to Germany and the time was constantly interrupted by technicalities like plane tickets, passports, and packing. I let myself read where my mood took me.

It took me into the home life of Augustus De Morgan. I had been working with this man long enough to know that he was a veritable fount of productivity. In my view he was not very inspired most of the time; there was no hope of finding sonorous sermons hidden in his works. But he was the father of a passel of children and still he wrote. He wrote and wrote and wrote. I was curious to know how he did it.

I looked in the *Memoir*, but in its pages children are given short shrift. The births of the last three girls go unrecorded; one of them, Anne, is never mentioned by name. The public life of Augustus as there constructed did not include children. It barely included Sophia either. "The great amount of work which he did," she wrote, "filled the day, so that I had but little of his society. We both naturally regretted this, but it could not be helped."

One of the few places Sophia admits irritation with her husband was in the context of vacations: "He bore a few weeks at Blackheath . . . but the heath, which he called a *desolation*, was a trial to him. After this summer he begged me to take the children without him; and I found that this arrangement, which I disliked, was the best." When Sophia and the children were at the beach, Augustus vacationed at home: "For myself, *solitude* is my relaxation," he confided to a friend. "When my family go away to the sea, and all the people leave town, and I sort all the letters, and put everything to rights, I feel what I used to hear called an *agreeable lull*." I could see how Augustus found time to write. But the answer did not satisfy me. I set out to find what I could about the author of this life.

In the only picture I could find, Sophia De Morgan cut a formidable figure. Seventy-six years old, swathed in widows' weeds, she is looking to the right of the photographer. One strong, capable hand emerges from her long black sleeve and rests on a book in her lap. Her face is strikingly unlined and calm. It is not at all hard to see through the effects of age the young woman she once was—strong, intelligent, with observing eyes and a sharp nose.

This picture forms the frontispiece of an autobiographical work Sophia was writing at the time of her death. I found it a frustrating read. Sophia so completely embraced her role as silent, invisible supporter to others that she barely appears in her own autobiography. The book is a long series of descriptions of important and interesting people she knew. But, she was a powerful person and at times, notably on the subject of children, her voice comes shining through.

> One day, when our conversation and our luncheon were finished at
> Upton House, Mrs. Fry's baby grandchild was bought in. Lady Byron,
> who was present, had a baby grandchild about the same age, and my
> own little one at home was not much older. I suppose we all mentally
> compared notes, and judging by myself, probably each one was quite
> certain that her baby far outshone the others in promise and beauty.

Sophia's "own little one" was at home for a reason; Alice was not always the clear winner of this kind of silent competition among women. Sophia goes on to describe another occasion in which she had brought her firstborn along.

> Little Alice, who had slept in the carriage the whole way, was far too
> wide awake when we were in Mrs. Baillie's drawing-room to sit quiet on

my knee and listen to the conversation. Everything in the room attracted her notice, and she wanted more attention than I could give, for she could run alone and talk at ten months old, and was a sweet and clever, but very excitable child. I heard afterwards that my friends thought my 'system of training' had been very faulty. If my baby had been properly managed from her birth, she would not have been so restless. I dare say they were in some measure right; any way, I have found some children so mercurial that nothing can make them quiet, steady characters; and some so heavy and dull that they cannot be roused into activity and interest.

It was intriguing to hear Sophia's approach to her children from a distance of almost fifty years, but in a biography of her son, the renowned ceramic artist William Frend De Morgan, I got a more direct view. There I found reprinted pieces of a nursery diary in which Sophia had conscientiously reported the ups and downs of life with her first babies: Alice, William, and George. The major force in the book is three-and-a-half-year-old Alice.

Alice was not what Sophia expected from a girl. She was constantly being reprimanded for not obeying orders until she knew the reasons behind them. She wiggled when the nurse tried to comb her hair.

Still, Sophia found much to be proud of in her busy daughter.

Willie, suffering from his teeth, was a little peevish yesterday when they were playing together. I said, "You don't mind it, do you, Allie, dear?"

"No," she said patronizingly. "It's his teeth you know. He's *irribubble!*"

Willie is much better [Sophia added a few days later]. He has just got a little gambroon dress and cape, trimmed with velvet and with silver buttons and buckle. This looks exceedingly nice and neat; and Alice and he were greatly delighted with it. I think it gave her as much pleasure to go to the drawer and look at Willie's new dress as if she had one herself.

Alice did not always find it easy to be Willy's sister, though, and as I tried in vain to concentrate on my proper work, I found the little girl's struggles to fit herself into the expectations of the world heartbreaking.

ALICE: "Mama, I wish I was not so contrairy."
MAMA: "Well, love, you will teach yourself in time not to be so."
ALICE: "Willy is good always."
MAMA: "Not quite always—but on the whole he is a dear good little boy."

ALICE: "He was born good—I wonder why I wasn't born good too. It was wrong in our Good Father—He ought to have borned me good too, ought not He?"

MAMA: "No—I do not think what He does is ever wrong. We cannot always tell *why* He does things different to what we wish, but we can know that if you had been born quite good, you would not have had the pleasure of conquering your naughtiness and of pleasing Him that way."

ALICE: "Then it was right in Him. *He done it to give me a job!*"

Alice was a handful, not just because of her behavior, but also because of her mind. "Alice calls the feathery white clouds 'the juice of the sky' because I had told her they were wet." Theological musings made especially good copy.

MAMA: "[God made the peach] and all the fruits that grow."

ALICE: "All fruits and trees and men and women and children. Everything but Himself. How *did* He come?—I cannot find out!"

MAMA: "No, you cannot—no one knows how He came."

ALICE: "For, you see, He could not make Himself because if He made Himself He must have had *arms* and if they were made He was made before He made Himself, and that could not be, you know."

Sophia was entranced by her daughter's intellectual wigglings, but Augustus was not. Sophia relates: "I must not conceal the fact that in the earlier part of his life he held man-like and masterful views of women's powers and privileges. Women, he thought, ought to have everything provided for them, and every trouble taken off their hands; so the less they meddled with business in any form the better. But these very young notions gave way, as he saw more of life, to wiser and more practical ones. He found that women were not utterly helpless, and his love of justice, combined with his better opinion of their powers, made him quite willing to concede to them as much as he would have desired for himself, namely, full scope and opportunity for the exercise of all their faculties." Whatever his mature opinions might have been, Augustus did not reach them before he and Sophia had clashed over Alice. "My eldest little girl gave alarming symptoms of being a prodigy," he wrote to a friend, "but I so effectually counteracted them that her mother began in her turn to be alarmed when she was between six and seven years old lest she should be backward in her learning."

Reading what little I could find about Alice rounded out the answer to my question about how Augustus could, for the most part, get on with his life undisturbed by complexities of family. It did not reassure me, though. I chafed under the restraints of my role as mother, restraints that kept me from sending my letter to Dr. Jennings. I chafed equally under the set of professional expectations that required me to keep working through Ned's illness. The positions defined by the two different roles I was expected to fill, mother and professor, were equally uncomfortable. De Morgan had defined them both, and neither was fair to the Alice in me.

I had loved my Cambridge office, but I was glad when the end of July meant I could stop pretending to work and unabashedly concentrate on my twentieth-century family which had again converged on Providence.

Ned's postsurgical appointment had been rescheduled for Wednesday, August 9. For two months I had been riding on the assumption that no news was good news, that the pathologist was correct in his preliminary conviction that Ned's tumor was benign. Now, finally, I was going to have a studied diagnosis.

"Neurosurgery. Dr. Jennings speaking."

"Oh, hello, Dr. Jennings. I was expecting to get Meghan. I was just calling to make sure you are having appointments today, before I brought Ned up to see you."

"Of course I have appointments today! I am seeing Ned."

"Fine, my second question is about the time of the appointment. Is it at twelve-thirty?"

"Yes, Mrs. Richards. That's right."

Ned and I had to park quite far away from the hospital, since the parking construction project blocked all nearby options. I tried to rush, but Ned's pace slowed inexorably the closer we got to the hospital. Dr. Jennings was looking over some files in the secretaries' office when Ned and I came in, flustered and about five minutes late. Before I could say a word he spoke.

"Mrs. Richards. I did not tell you twelve-thirty. I just said the appointment was *today*. It's at four."

I almost retorted, but I caught myself in time: Joan, it is not your job to tell this guy how to behave. "OK. We can go to the museum and come back then."

"Oh, no, you don't need to do that! I can fit you in now."

I couldn't believe this. Why had he gone to the trouble of telling me I was wrong if it didn't matter? "Fine," I said, as cooperatively as I could.

Dr. Jennings beckoned us into his office.

"Edward, let's see that scar. . . . Look's good. And how are you feeling? . . . Great. Vision good? . . . Wonderful. . . ."

The surgeon turned to me. "Mrs. Richards, he seems fine. The pathologists confirmed that the tumor was a pylocitic astrocytoma with no other cells mixed in. This is very good news. This kind doesn't come back. You will need to get an MRI for him after six months and after a year. But my previous recommendation of one every three months is unnecessary. This kind does not come back."

"Thank God! *What* good news!"

"Yes, it is. And this is a good day!" Dr. Jennings accompanied us to the door. "Did you see the girl who came in just before you? I operated on her eight years ago! And earlier today there was a boy I operated on eleven years ago! And now Edward! It makes me feel like a father."

There was a tiny hesitancy behind the statement that gave me pause. This man has been operating on patients at the rate of three or four a week for at least fifteen years. To see three that he thinks will survive constitutes a red-letter day. "You do good work, Dr. Jennings," I said, wanting to reassure him.

Part II
Beim Wippen
(On a See-Saw)

Once a boy on a German Class trippe
Fell terribly hard from a *Wippe**
They cut his arm open
And found it was broken
Then sewed it so it wouldn't rippe.

(Ned Richards)

* A *Wippe* (pronounced *vippa*) is a common piece of German playground
equipment that is basically a see-saw with springs.

Berlin

On August 15 we flew to Berlin. By the time we actually got into the plane, for Rick and me the adventure was as much about escape as about exploring new horizons. The apparently positive outcome of the surgery was an infinite blessing, but even it had been slow in coming.

The move was something else again for the children. For Brady it was blessed action after a long, hot, and idle summer. Too old for summer camp, too young for a summer job, he was glad by August to have any excuse to do something other than lie around his room. As for the larger issue of a year abroad, Brady was old enough to see the power of an abstract rationale; as he put it: "I do not want to leave Providence, but I can see it will be good for me."

Ned, for his part, was considerably less receptive to a move that would separate him from his familiar haunts. I had initially expected my ever-curious and adventurous little boy to be excited by the thought of a faraway land with a new and exotic language. In the event, he preferred his adventures in the world of *Dungeons and Dragons* or *Magic* cards. He was deeply grounded in a particular place and had no desire to explore the exotica of Germany. His resistance was immediate and loudly voiced as soon as we announced our intention of going; the medical saga that dominated the intervening time did plenty to augment and nothing to diminish it.

The move had a real downside for Rick and me as well. Rick had realized, sometime in April, that his hopes of leaving his job for a year to come with us were unrealistic. In a period of cost-cutting he did not dare take a leave of absence from the State Department of Education. For my part, however, it was almost a necessity to take the fellowship. Our year coping with Ned's tumor had taken a large bite of time from my book. There was no place for excuses and I desperately needed unencumbered time to concentrate on the project wholeheartedly. To those who asked why I would go to Germany to write a book on Victorian England I replied from a Newtonian point of view in which the particularities of time and place are ultimately trivial. Triangles and clocks are the same in Berlin as in London or Providence; nothing essential separates one location from another. The Berlin fellowship promised me time, and that was ultimately real: I could not afford to let it go.

Rick and I had never been apart for more than a few weeks in our twenty-five-year marriage, but we comforted ourselves with the example of friends who had negotiated commuting relationships for years. It was not what any of us wanted, but we were clear about what we were doing. Rick was taking a month to help us all to settle in. In addition he had already reserved a series of tickets for weeklong sojourns that extended into April.

The *Wissenschaftskolleg* sent a secretary to meet our sleepy, jet-lagged family and drive us to the apartment where the boys and I were to spend the year. Exhausted though we were, the situation in which we found ourselves woke us all up instantly. We were to be housed in a veritable castle, the Villa Walther, built by a Russian prince early in the century. Statuary covered its façade, a frieze decorated the peak of the roof, Latin quotations and Roman medallions were scattered randomly across its front. In the back, the building formed a U around a terrace and fishpond, complete with fish and water lilies, though not a great deal of water. A host of naked cherubs supported a second-floor balcony; two concrete Roman soldiers with metal spears stood guard over a double set of steps leading away.

Beyond was a large yard, technically a small park, or *Grünanlage,* with a rose garden, an unexplained granite obelisk topped by a metal ball, and a terrace with a couple of benches. The terrace overlooked a small lake, or *See,* one of a chain of four on which the Villa Walther was situated. Underneath the terrace was a grottoed boathouse. Within minutes of our arrival we were accosted by an outgoing fellow, anxious to sell us a share in a small rowboat. It was the perfect first step toward reconciling Ned to his new abode.

The apartment itself was on the second floor of the lake side of the U. This was a five-story, modern reconstruction of a previously destroyed wing. On one side of the living room/kitchen area of the apartment a small balcony overlooked a wooded area and canal. On the other side windows looked out into a tangle of open-air balcony-hallways that lined the inside of the U. Brady's room overlooked the gorge from one side of the living room, mine did the same from the other. Ned's bedroom faced the inner courtyard on a level with the balcony-supporting cherubs. Brady had his own half-bath; a large full bath lay between Ned's and my rooms.

The living room was furnished with a brown couch and two easy chairs. They were huge and oddly amorphous; heavy padding slumped formless over some deeply hidden inner structure. They were comfortable in a somewhat decadent way, but hardly perky. There was not much else by way of décor and not a great deal of light; we were at the bottom of a large building. The corridors impeded light into the courtyard windows, and, on the other side, the gorge was choked with trees. Still, none of us has ever lived in a place even remotely so exotic and I suspect that none of us ever will again. For a year's sabbatical adventure, the dark apartment in the Villa Walther was just fine.

The city in which we found ourselves promised to be everything we had hoped and more: large, cosmopolitan, blessed with numerous green areas and amazingly conflict-free to American eyes. The public veneer of commerce—movies, advertisements, offerings of the shops—were surprisingly and, to Ned at least, comfortingly familiar. The images often were the same, and virtually everyone spoke English well enough to accommodate our linguistic failures. Brady was at first disappointed in his hopes of finding an exotic new culture: after a couple of hours casing out the shops on the major commercial street, the Kufürstendamm, he opined, "It's just like any big American city, only in German."

Over the course of the next few days, however, we modified this assessment. We had expected and found that we could get virtually anywhere in the city on public transport, and we basked in the freedom of an efficient, safe transportation system. We quickly discovered the Number 119 bus, which picked us up a block from the Villa Walther and then rolled up the Kurfürstendamm, the main street of erstwhile West Berlin. Berliner buses are huge double-decker affairs that lumber through the streets extraordinarily on time. The first level is utilitarian, with the driver, some seating, and areas for luggage, wheelchairs, and strollers. We preferred the second level, up a small circular staircase behind the driver. There the ceiling is low but the view privileged. When front seats were free, we chose them; with lots of legroom facing a huge wraparound front window, they felt like a mobile living room.

In our first couple of days we located appropriate grocery stores along the 119 bus route. By Saturday we were ready for a more substantial expedition. Our goal was an English bookstore that Rick had found in our little guidebook. It was all very well that Germans spoke English in the streets, but at home we needed reading material. We studied our map and planned a route down the increasingly familiar Kurfürstendamm, changing at the downtown zoo to the 100 bus that would take us to the bookstore. The plan had the added feature that the 100 bus route was a veritable tourist heaven, passing all sorts of key places in Berlin's fractured twentieth-century past. It seemed the perfect outing, and by eleven o'clock Rick and I had herded the boys out into the warm sunny day.

We rolled with our 119 bus past the top of the Kurfürstendamm and got off in an open square with a subway station: Wittenbergplatz. To the side was a sign—*Orte des Schreckens, die wir niemals vergessen dürfen*—from which hung a series of place names: Auschwitz, Stutthof, Daidanek, Treblinka, Theresienstadt, Buchenwald, Dachau, Sachsenhausen, Ravensbrück, Bergen-Belsen, Trostencz, Flossenbürg. I puzzled out its meaning: "Places of horror that we must never forget." The names were the destinations to which Jews had been sent from the Wittenbergplatz subway station. The city bustled around us with commercial uncaring, but on me the memorial worked its desired effect, and I found the place to be very unsettling.

We walked down the street toward the huge, *Gedächnis Kirche,* or memorial church, the beautifully preserved, bombed-out ruin of a late nineteenth-century cathedral. Street musicians, sidewalk artists, beggars, and magicians competed for our attention in a large open square. We bought bratwurst from a pushcart vendor and moseyed about, looking at people and into elegant shop windows.

Then we located and boarded the 100 bus bound for the English bookstore. The second tier was hot but the view was stimulating and our fellow passengers cheerful. Ned and Rick got two front seats; Brady and I sat behind.

"*Gucke mal! Gucke mal!* Look! Look!" a little girl insisted to her mother. "*Das Schloss Bellevue. Gucke mal!* The Castle Bellevue. Look!"

Brady and I followed her pointing finger to the pretty castle. For a moment I wondered what kind of education could instill such historical/architectural interest in a child of five. Then I saw the naked man strolling down the path toward the bus.

"Oh, Dad! Will they arrest him?" Ned asked in great excitement.

"Shut up, Ned!" Brady commanded, blushing.

"I doubt it, Ned," Rick answered. "Being naked is not such a big deal in Germany."

Brady turned to me and changed the subject. "What does '*Gucke mal!*' mean?" he asked.

"I guess it means 'Look!'" I said.

"'*Gucke mal!*'" he practiced under his breath.

"But you'd better be careful with it," I went on. "It was a little girl talking to her mother. I don't know whether it is something you would say to a teacher, for example."

"I *know* that, Mom."

The bus went on, past the Reichstag, the German parliament building. The artist Christo had wrapped it in July; we missed seeing his work by only two weeks. Now the whole enormous structure was surrounded by empty scaffolding, and by plywood walls plastered with posters describing the major renovation project to prepare the building to be again the seat of German government.

Then, on the left, was the *Brandenburger Tor*, the Brandenburg gate, huge, implacable, the horses and chariot on its top thundering ahead of us. "The Kaiser was a very bad man, Joan. He tried to take over all of Europe, even England." Grandmama's voice echoed in my ears. Our bus made a quick turn through the portal and into a different world—East Berlin, or at least it was called that until six years before, when it was part of East Germany. Now it was no longer communist, the border no longer sealed. But the street vendors in the square behind the gate were hawking Russian nesting dolls. As the bus moved along I felt a frisson of fear and wished I had brought our passports. We got off at the first stop.

Nobody got off of the bus with us. As we stood, virtually alone, on the large and basically deserted boulevard, I was acutely aware that this had also been the downtown of Hitler's Berlin, that his administration had once worked out of the buildings all around us. They were huge, stone, and apparently empty. Everything was gray and dusty. The sun was hot. We consulted our map; the bookstore should be a few blocks away.

We set off down a side street. The dark buildings came right to the sidewalks. Pieces of paper blew in the street. Ned began to whine. "I'm hot, Dad. Can't we go home?"

Nervousness made Rick edgy. "Hush up, Ned. We are going to the bookstore! We need to get books. We can't go through another week with nothing to read!"

We walked a block. The corner just revealed more of the same in all four directions. We went on, silent. The buildings became ever more sinister; they breathed a mixture of Nazi hate and East German despair. At about the same moment Brady and I focused on the nicks and holes in the building stones.

"Are these bullet holes?" he asked.

"I think so," I replied.

The next corner opened somewhat—there was a strange fifties' kind of building, a deserted park, an *U-Bahn,* or subway, station. Beyond was a vacant lot. We kept going. Most of the next block was under construction. None of the several construction machines was in operation; I would have welcomed their movement to offset the singularity of ours. We clattered through plywood tunnels designed to protect us from falling debris. We saw a street sign, consulted our map, and pressed on; just one more block. We looked for numbers—48, 50, and now 52. There was no sign, but the English titles on the books in the window indicated that we had reached our destination. What a relief!

Just as we were turning into the door a woman came briskly out of it. We stepped aside to let her by, but instead she turned to lock it.

"Excuse me, but we wanted to go in" Rick said in polite disbelief.

"I'm sorry," she replied. "It's two o'clock! Closing time!"

We were taken aback. It would have been nice if the place had advertised their truncated hours in the guide book.

"Next week is long Saturday. We are open until four then."

"Oh, can't you just let us buy a book?" I begged internally, but I was being silly. We had arrived too late.

But as we retraced our steps to the Villa Walther we found ourselves moving through a virtual ghost town. Only then did we realize that, by law, *all* stores were closed by two o'clock on Saturday and all day Sunday. Fortunately we had enough food to carry us through some kind of patchwork supper when we got home. Even more fortunately, the only person I knew in Berlin had invited us for brunch on Sunday. We arrived a famished foursome and left with begged dinner-makings. Berlin was not "just like any big American city, only in German."

Verlezt (Injured)

Within a week of our arrival, school started. Rick and I had decided to send the boys to the bilingual John F. Kennedy School, in the heart of what had been the American sector of Berlin. Until the fall of the wall, the English-speaking part of the student body had been predominantly the children of the occupying army. Soon it was to be the bastion of embassy children who would be in Berlin in force when the capital moved from Bonn. Now it was in transition, and the students were culled from a wide variety of backgrounds and circumstances.

The trip to school began with a fifteen-minute walk along a wooded path beside the waters of a placid *See* behind the Villa Walther. We watched the ducks, particularly charmed by the pert little Muscovy ones that came for the winter. There was also a lone heron who could be counted on to be perched, one-legged, on a favorite rock. Just after we passed the heron, the path went up, and we climbed out of the woods a block from the stop for the 110 bus.

The bus was full of schoolchildren, pushing to get up the little stairs, standing, sitting, jabbering, knapsacks on their backs. Ned and I found a seat on the unpopular first level; Brady and Rick stood. I tried to make conversation with Ned but was quickly put down. "Shhh, Mom! They'll know we don't speak German." So I sat quietly and took in the scenes along the route.

The bus rumbled through miles of posh residences. At one point, we passed an elaborate, red brick *Rathaus,* or city hall. Then, after another mile or two of residences, a large working farm unfolded on the other side of the bus. I nudged Ned and pointed. The farm stopped and the bus went on, past more houses. Then we came to the American embassy, surrounded by barbed wire and fairly bristling with defenses. Acres of deserted army barracks sprawled around it and across the street. The bus turned left onto a major boulevard and left the embassy behind. A wooded campus of stucco buildings labeled itself: *Otto-Hoffen-Heim, Orthopädisches Krankenhaus* [Orthopedic Hospital]. More residences, a commercial area, on the other side of the bus a park, and then, the John F. Kennedy School. The trip took about thirty minutes.

The school counselor introduced Brady to a student sponsor and they disappeared into the high school; he directed Ned, Rick, and me in another direction to find Ned's class, with "Mrs. Harkin in Red, 305." We were soon lost in a maze of doors and corridors so we stopped a couple of children to ask for directions. "Red, 305? Oh that's just up these stairs and through the red doors. . . . *Hallo Gerhardt! Wie geht's?*" and they jabbered off in German. We went up the green stairs and through the red-framed glass doors to Room 305.

Mrs. Harkin was as American and as tall as I, head topped by thick, decidedly white hair. She didn't need to tell us she had been teaching for over twenty years. She was the sharp, clear essence of an elementary school teacher. Ned was in very good hands. He emerged at the end of the day, amazed and energized.

"The kids all speak German *and* English. They're better than the teachers. The gym teacher can't speak English at all. And Mr. Arnold's German is worse than yours, Mom. But the kids just switch. Like a radio station. Mrs. Harkin says if I work at it, I could learn to be that way, too."

Brady explored on his own, but for the first several days, Rick and/or I accompanied Ned to and from school. It was not a bad trip, but by the end of the week, making it twice a day became more disruptive than interesting. We were glad as Ned got more confident and recognized the crucial stops. I made up a packet with identification and a bit of emergency money and we left him to make his own way on the bus with the crowds of Berlin's other schoolchildren.

A few days after we decided he could cope, Ned got home frightened, almost an hour later than usual. He had taken a wrong bus that did not make the full run but instead stopped for good at the American Embassy corner.

"It wasn't even a regular stop, Mom! It was all turned around! I sat there, but then the bus driver yelled at me in German so I had to get off."

"Oh dear, sweetie! Then what did you do?"

"Well, I thought I would have to walk home. But then I crossed the street to the side where the regular buses go. I found a bus stop that said 110, and another bus came and I took it." As he tearfully told his tale, Ned began to see its other side. He had been thwarted and found his way home. The Berlin transportation system never again held any fears for him.

Mastering transportation was an important step toward Ned's and my freedom from each other. Another part of the plan involved after-school programs. Most German children get out of school at noon to be home in time for lunch; one of the features of the Kennedy School was that the boys had lunch at school and the day wasn't over until two o'clock. That was better than noon, but even with a forty-minute trip home there was still a long and lonely afternoon to fill.

There were a number of after-school programs among which to choose, though, and Ned and I decided on the swim team for him. The team practiced two or three times a week in the pool of the old American army compound on the 110 bus route. They had a long and intriguing schedule of meets culminating in a national competition in Munich. Ned's scar showed clearly through his wet hair as he swam vigorously and well for the tryouts. He was one of only three fifth graders accepted directly onto the team. I signed up to assist the coach on Saturdays and Ned and I went home triumphant. Berlin was becoming ever more interesting to Ned and manageable to me.

As the boys became more integrated at school, I wondered about the right time to inform Ned's teachers about his medical past. His scar was daily becoming more hidden in his rapidly growing hair and he displayed it only as social capital among his peers. I believed his seizures were a closed book, but Dr. Gasparian would not confirm my conviction. He had pronounced Ned's postsurgical EEG "fine for someone who just had neurosurgery," and kept him firmly on Tegretol for at least a year. I did not want Ned's new school to regard him as strange or frightening but it would certainly be irresponsible not to inform them of his situation. After a couple of days I sat down and told the basic story to his homeroom teacher, Mrs. Harkin, and to Frau Kindl, the secretary who doubled as a nurse. It was a relief to get it off my mind and neither woman seemed concerned that the school could not handle the situation.

Weekends remained a challenge. They began crisply, with a full-family forced march to get groceries. After this burst of activity, however, we faced an action vacuum. Brady was quite content to cocoon in his room, but Ned poured all of his resentments about having been uprooted into the empty days. I was always ready for a trip to a museum or some historical site, but Ned did not share my enthusiasms.

More successful were Rick's trips to the movies. I hated going to the glitzy Americanized theaters at the top of the Kurfürstendamm. There the offerings *were* just the same as in America only in German. But the men in my life were intrigued and emerged grinning from movies they had seen before in English. Random German phrases emerged from these outings and were sprinkled through otherwise mundane conversations. *Spinst du?* Are you crazy? *Quatsch!* Nonsense! *Keine Bewegung!* Freeze!

As the boys settled into school I began to figure out my academic landscape. My year at the Dibner had promised a year of intense sholarship, but the strain of Ned's medical problems had meant that I did not really take advantage of it. Dr. Jennings's assurance, "this kind doesn't come back," was the promise of a clean slate.

The *Wissenschaftskolleg* was imposing and empty. We had come early to accommodate the boys' school year; the other fellows were not due to arrive until mid-October. But within two weeks of my arrival I found the *Max Planck Institut für Wissenschaftsgeschichte*, the Max Planck Institute for the History of Science. The Max Planck was located in the former Czech embassy in the *Mitte*, or middle of Berlin. The first time I visited, about a week after our arrival, I recognized the building as the 1950s structure we had passed on our aborted trip to the English bookstore.

I went there first to talk with Genie, who was beginning her first year as its director. Genie is one of my best friends in the world. I met her first in graduate school. At first all of the graduate students moved more or less together, but after the first year we began to concentrate on our own specialties. The others would come to me for information, for answers when their work abutted mine, but, for the most part, they had no desire to join me among my mathematicians. They stopped listening long before I had developed the full extent of what I had been concentrating on, just as I stopped listening to them as they rode their particular hobbyhorses into intellectual thickets.

It was here that Genie was different. She was interested in the same things I was. She was always ready to meet me at the outermost edges of my thinking, she was always ready to help me when I got stuck, she was always ready to rejoice when I made a breakthrough. As long as Genie was there I never really worked alone.

Upon graduation, Genie and I had gone in different directions. I was at the time already nine years into my marriage, ready for children, and some semblance of settled family life. Genie was still single and more restless. Her star climbed meteorically from one prestigious position to another. Along the way she had married a German and their paths led her to Berlin. Like many people in small fields, I am the only historian of science at Brown, and I often find it intellectually lonely. A large part of the attraction of my fellowship year was the lure of a year again working close to Genie.

When I arrived in Berlin, Genie's special gift for intellectual communication was being embodied in the odd building in the *Mitte* that housed her institute. As August moved into September, the fellows of the Max Planck Institute were beginning to gather. A few I knew well: Liza was another friend from graduate school, who was there for the fall, finishing a book with Genie, and there was Snorri, an Icelandic man who worked with our advisor about five years behind us. Most were people I'd known only through their work. There was Clare, whose work on women in science had long fascinated me, but whom I'd met only briefly here and there. There was Rudolf, a German, who was just back from several years in Cambridge, England, where he investigated the work of Victorian physicists. There was Plato, a Dutchman, whose work on probability theory complemented mine. And there were others, including a number of younger German and American postdoctorates, as yet new to me. It was exciting to interact with the group fast gathering in Berlin. I was well on my way to figuring out the mechanics of the boys' school lives. Then I could enter the world of scholarship again, not forever, but for a blessed year.

The recognition of how short that time was, combined with the initial headiness of renewed contact with people who saw the value of my work, spurred me into my small office in the deserted *Kolleg*. The weather in this early September was warm and muggy; I had the building to myself, and I left several doors open to create a draft. Rick was down the street in the small apartment, doing some of his work on the dining room table. It was a nagging reality that he would not be there much longer, but on this September morning it was still almost a week until he would be gone. Like the grasshopper who fiddled into the fall, I felt no need to miss him yet.

I began to get organized, unpacking my standard texts for reference. As I plodded through the boring process I noticed Newton's *Principia,* and mused about the kinds of thinking that somehow made this whole extraordinary German adventure of ours possible.

Absolute, true, and mathematical time. . .
Absolute space, in its own nature. . .
Place is a part of space which a body takes up . . .
Positions properly have no quantity. . .

It was thirty years since I'd first encountered Newton's rolling balls. Now I was once again in a rather small room, though this one was bright and sunny. Newton's ball, however, was unaffected. It rolled through my open door, past the desk, out the open window and across the hot and muggy German street as calmly as ever. Eternal, infinite, everywhere present, Newton's absolute space lay open behind all the apparent newness of my situation.

It was interesting to contemplate all of this from Berlin, though. The city that surrounded me had been the home of Gottfried Wilhelm Leibniz, one of Newton's arch-rivals in both mathematics and philosophy. In the first decades of the eighteenth century Newton was President of the Royal Society and the Master of the Mint. Leibniz, for his part, was the founder of the Berlin Academy and philosopher in the court of Sophia Charlotte, the wife of Friedrich I, the first king of Prussia. From these rather different but equally well-established positions the two men battled over which of them deserved the credit for having developed the calculus first.

I have never been particularly interested in questions of priority, but the differences between Newton and Leibniz were more interesting than that. The depth and breadth of their disagreement is reflected in a correspondence that Leibniz initiated in 1715. In November of that year he wrote a letter to the Princess of Wales, Caroline of Ansbach. He knew her well. She was a German princess who was orphaned from the age of twelve and grew up in the court of Sophia Charlotte. Sophia Charlotte loved the little girl as her own and gave Leibniz the task of educating the young Caroline. Years passed, Caroline grew up and got married, and then the vagaries of royal succession had made her husband, Georg Augustus of Hanover, next in line for the British throne. So he and Caroline went to England anticipating the moment (it came in 1727) when he would become King George II and she his queen.

Caroline was a strong-minded and intelligent woman, but Leibniz feared that in England she would fall under Newton's sway. "Natural religion itself, seems to decay (in England) very much. Many will have human souls to be material: others make God himself a corporeal being," he warned. He cited as central evidence of this dangerous materialism Newton's statement that "space is the sensorium of God." God does not stand "in need of any organ to perceive things by," Leibniz insisted.

Caroline showed Leibniz's letter to Samuel Clarke, the avowed Newtonian minister of her new English court. "[He] is not willing to admit that Mr. Newton has the opinions which you ascribe to him," she explained in a letter containing Clarke's rebuttal of Leibniz's charges. "He shows a great desire to convict me of holding wrong opinions, but in vain," Leibniz replied. And so it went, back and forth, until Leibniz died a year later. By that time the German had written five letters and the Englishman had responded to them all.

The driving force behind the correspondence was theological, but the letters moved freely across fields we would distinguish as philosophy and physics as well. For the eighteenth-century participants there was little difference among them. This did not just reflect an eclectic vision, it affected the very terms of the argument, the criteria by which a position was considered valid or not. "I could not help myself saying to Dr. Clarke that your opinion seems the more conformable to the perfection of God and that any philosophy which would lead me away from it appears to me imperfect," Caroline affirmed to Leibniz, "since in my opinion philosophy was made, or ought to be sought, in order to make us more tranquil in spirit and to strengthen us against ourselves and against everything outside us which may assail us, and I cannot believe it could have this effect if it showed us the imperfection of God."

Leibniz agreed, and for him Newton's views of time and space constituted just such a threat to philosophical/theological tranquility. In his view Newton's absolute space implied "the imperfection of God" because it created choices that even God could not reasonably make. "Supposing any one should ask, why God did not create everything a year sooner; and the same person should infer from thence, that God has done something, concerning which 'tis not possible there should be a reason, why he did it so, and not otherwise: and the answer is that his inference would be right." Newton's spatial and temporal absolutes were simply too huge and undifferentiated. In the face of such immensity, such eternity, even God would have no way of knowing where or when to begin.

So, Leibniz insisted, there is no absolute space, no absolute time. "As for my own opinion," he wrote, "I hold space to be something merely relative, as time is; . . . For space denotes, in terms of possibility, an order to things which exist at the same time, considered as existing together; . . . And when many things are seen together, one perceives that order of things among themselves."

The exchange of letters was terminated by Leibniz's death, which seems somehow symbolic of the outcome of the philosophical discussion. By its end the Princess of Wales was moving toward the English side; certainly the larger world of Western Europe moved in that direction, and by the middle of the eighteenth century Leibniz's physical ideas were all but forgotten. Physics on the continent was thoroughly Newtonian and it remained that way for a century and a half. It was not until Einstein developed his ideas at the beginning of the twentieth century that anyone again seriously challenged Newton's absolute time and space.

As I pawed through the crates of books in my *Wissenschaftskolleg* study I mused about the ways in which Newtonian thinking somehow made the whole extraordinary German adventure of ours possible. Any world in which it was simply accepted that I could move my family 4,000 miles and set up shop in Berlin was a world deeply grounded in the essentially Newtonian supposition that place has no real importance, that "positions properly have no quantity."

The phone rang. I started. Who do I know in Berlin? How do I answer the phone in German? The phone rang again.

"Hello. This is Joan Richards."

"Hello, Mrs. Richards. This is Frau Kindl, the nurse at the John F. Kennedy School. Your son, Ned, . . ."

How much can one think or feel in the nanosecond between an introduction and the completion of the sentence? How much of a year's frantic anxiety and fear can be recalled before the next words are registered?

"Your son, Ned, says he is feeling dizzy and wants to go home."

"Your son, Ned, says he can't see very well. He seems to have a terrible headache. Can you come and bring him home?"

"Your son, Ned, has had some kind of fit. Come immediately; he is unconscious. We have called an ambulance and he is on his way to . . ."

I held the phone and watched myself holding the phone; I listened and listened to myself listening. "Your son, Ned, fell in the park. His arm is hurting him a great deal. We think it may be broken."

"He fell in the park, the playground?" I repeated tentatively. Was there no seizure, nothing more than an injured arm? "Where is he now?" I asked.

"Oh, he is here, in my office," she said. "He is lying down. I do not want to send him to his classroom until a doctor has looked at this arm, though. I think it might be broken."

I reentered my body and the conversation. "It will take me a little while to get there," I said, as I planned my route. "Tell him it will be about an hour."

"OK," she agreed. "But do come as soon as you can. His arm seems quite painful."

I couldn't have been less perturbed as I hung up the phone and set out to collect Rick. It was so normal, so manageable—a broken arm. Rick was equally serene as we made our way to the school. "It's probably not even broken," we agreed. "Probably he fell, cried, and then had to justify his tears. He has spent so much time with doctors recently that he feels almost safest in a medical situation. It's probably nothing at all."

When we got to the school we found Ned lying on a couch, clutching his left arm tightly to his chest. It was very swollen and obviously very painful. Ned was not just being dramatic; a doctor was in order.

Frau Kindl was glad to see us. When we admitted we had not yet been even a month in Berlin and had no idea of how to handle a medical situation she offered two options: either we could go a couple of miles up the road to the Otto-Hoffen-Heim, the orthopedic teaching hospital of the *Freie Universität* [Free University], or we could go just down the street to a private *Arzt*, a doctor, Dr. Schwalbach. He was comfortable speaking English, had a solid practice that included his own X-ray machine, and had worked with children from the school for years. Many parents found it easier to work with a single practitioner than to try to negotiate the complexities of a full-blown hospital for something as straightforward as a playground injury.

The thought of a hospital was simply horrible to both Rick and me. We carefully but cheerfully maneuvered Ned into a makeshift splint and got into the cab that would take us to see Dr. Schwalbach. It appeared that our Berlin adventure was going to have a medical chapter, but in this area we had certainly seen it all. After a brain tumor, a broken arm held no particular fears for us.

Kontrolle (Checking)

Dr. Schwalbach's office was on the first floor of a gray Berlin apartment building. From the inside, though, it looked and felt reassuringly medical. The walls were white, and a couple of white-clad receptionists looked up expectantly as we came in. Language was a problem but we struggled along in whichever worked for the moment, registering Ned and clarifying his insurance. The latter was a cause for rejoicing. Because Ned's tumor constituted a preexisting condition we had kept our insurance policy in the states. But our health maintenance organization was so totally unprepared to deal with new situations that might develop overseas that just seven days before we had bought a German policy to deal with immediate problems. A simple telephone call confirmed that care for Ned's arm would be paid for, and the subject never arose again.

Ned gripped his arm to his chest as these questions were settled. Then, before we had time to take a seat in the waiting room, a blond, bespectacled man, somewhere in his early forties, appeared from down the hall. "*Hallo*," he said to Ned and to us. The adults shook hands; Ned clutched his arm.

Dr. Schwalbach turned his attention to the immediate problem. He looked respectfully at the swollen arm and hesitated to touch it. Instead he questioned Ned to ascertain that it was painful if moved but all right if held tight. "We take an X ray," he said and Ned was turned over to one of the nurses.

The woman was efficient, but the process was difficult. The doctor wanted one picture of Ned's arm when bent, which was not a problem, but straightening it for the other picture was agony. Ned screamed as the nurse forced it open on the table. She ran to take the picture, then immediately gave him permission to bend and hold it again. Rick and I heard the drama from outside the room; both Ned and the nurse emerged somewhat shaken but having followed directions. Rick held Ned close to him in the waiting room as the pictures were developed. The arm did seem to be badly hurt.

But when the X rays appeared, they were completely clean. Dr. Schwalbach poured over them and could find nothing wrong; he showed them to me and we scrutinized them together. An X ray of an arm has a completely different emotional impact than does an MRI of the brain; I looked with irrational pride at the straight unblemished bones that lay hidden in Ned's arm.

"Could it be a problem with the cartilage?" I asked. "Something with the epiphyses?" I went on, proud to know the technical term for the growth point of a child's bones. Dr. Schwalbach said "perhaps" and took another set of pictures of Ned's right arm to see whether comparative differences showed up. He poured over both sets of X rays but found nothing. "*Starke Prellung*" [badly bruised], he wrote in Ned's computer records. Rick and I grinned with relief—Ned would probably be swimming again within two weeks.

A nurse made a splint for Ned, bound his arm to it with an Ace bandage, and made a sling to support the whole. He tentatively trusted his arm to this apparatus and let his right arm drop as he walked down the hall from the nurse's workroom. "Don't walk around with the splint more than you have to," Dr. Schwalbach said. "Be still and hold the arm above your heart as much as you can. Come back tomorrow morning."

Rick and I took Ned home on the *S-Bahn*, or surface rail, and laid him on the couch. We propped the arm on pillows and surrounded it with bags of frozen peas. Ned occasionally cried out in spontaneous pain while we read to him.

The next morning we again set out. Gingerly we wended our way through the hour of public transportation that separated us by an hour from Dr. Schwalbach. He gently unwrapped Ned's arm, looked at it, wrote "*Kontrolle*" [checking] in the computer record, and wrapped it up again. When I brought up the problem of pain, the doctor suggested Tylenol but declined to prescribe anything stronger. "Come back tomorrow," he said.

"Tomorrow" was Saturday, and Dr. Schwalbach was not in his office. Instead we were greeted by a Rumanian doctor, Schwalbach's *Kollege*, who spoke no English. We limped along in German. I again explained that Ned was in considerable pain; the doctor seemed more receptive than Dr. Schwalbach had been and gave us a prescription. "*Kommen Sie Montag zurück*. Come back on Monday," he said.

It was a wonderful surprise to find that the prescription was free from the *Apotheke*. It was less wonderful to find, after pouring over the accompanying literature, that it was for Tylenol suppositories, and that the dosage prescribed was that for a six-year-old. I went back to giving

Ned the over-the-counter pills he was used to, in the dosage suggested for his age group.

By Monday, Ned's arm was still very swollen but becoming less painful. I thought he was ready to go back to school. Again we journeyed across town to the office of Dr. Schwalbach. Again he unwrapped the arm. "Come back tomorrow" he said, as he wrote "*Kontrolle*" in Ned's file.

I began to see a double meaning to these *Kontrollen.* Initially it had been reassuring that Dr. Schwalbach was willing to take Ned's elbow seriously enough to monitor it daily, but at this point it did not seem to warrant the effort. Tuesday was a very busy day. Rick was flying back to his job in Rhode Island and I wanted the time to see him off. The two hours on public transport that were involved in getting to Dr. Schwalbach seemed long and unnecessary. But when I explained my busy morning to him, he responded simply, "Come in the afternoon."

We came the following afternoon, after school. By this time Ned and I were used to the basic procedure at Dr. Schwalbach's. We did not have a fixed appointment, but simply came in the afternoon office hours. Within half an hour we would be called and directed to a tiny examining room—one of a row in the back of Dr. Schwalbach's offices. There we would sit listening as Dr. Schwalbach made his way towards us. "*So . . . Edward . . .*" he would greet Ned in German as he came in. He would stretch the phrase long enough to make the linguistic switch. "How is your arm?" Then he would unwrap the arm and look at it. This Tuesday afternoon we were rewarded. Ned's arm seemed less swollen and painful. Dr. Schwalbach wrote "*Deutlich besser*" [clearly better] in his computer file and took away the sling; I felt *deutlich besser* as well when he allowed us two days before the next appointment.

"*Auf Wiedersehen,*" the people in the waiting room would say as we left.

On Thursday, a week after the initial fall, Dr. Schwalbach removed the splint. Ned was intrigued as he looked at his arm but surprised to find that he could not move it at all. He did not try very hard, because it was still very painful. Dr. Schwalbach rewrapped the arm in an Ace bandage, but Ned was not comfortable. Surprised, the doctor gave Ned the splint to wear if he wanted; he again allowed us two days before the next appointment.

By the time we had made our way home, Ned definitely wanted the splint. I replaced it, he immediately felt better, and we did not take it off again. At the Saturday appointment, however, Schwalbach's *Kollege* was not pleased. He took the splint away and firmly told Ned "*Sei tapfer!* Be brave!" Ned looked wispy with pain. He clutched his arm to his chest as we walked out into the warm fall day. I did not tell him what *Sei tapfer* meant.

The rest of the morning was taken up with expeditions on various forms of transport to lay in food for the weekend if not the week. Ned straggled along while Brady and I made forays into various shops and struggled to carry our purchases home. By the early afternoon everything was closed and the challenge changed dramatically. There was nothing more to do until Monday morning.

Lunch was quiet. Rick's absence hung heavy upon the three of us.

"I want Dad!" The desire exploded angrily out of Ned. Realizing what he had said, he was overwhelmed by its truth. "I want Dad! I want my father! I want Dad!" he sobbed, holding his injured arm against him.

"Oh, Ned! Don't be so dumb!" Brady retorted. "Dad isn't here! Grow up!" He stalked to his room.

"Neddy, come here." I settled myself receptively on the couch.

"I don't want to come there! I don't want to sit with you! I want my *Dad!*"

"Shut up, Ned!" Brady yelled from his room.

Ned went down the hall to Brady's room. Disaster loomed. But the boys recognized their common lot. The yelling ceased and they spent the afternoon playing cards as far as possible from my perch in the living room. Berlin is 4,000 miles from Providence.

"I'm sorry about Dad," I said as I tucked Ned in that night. "I miss him too."

"Mom, my arm hurts." He changed the subject.

"I'm sorry about that too. I think it will be better soon, though."

Sunday dawned, sunny, pleasant, and new. During my solitary Saturday I had wrestled with a German guidebook and hit upon the *Pfaueninsel,* or Peacock's Island, as a promising destination for a picnic. In addition to free-ranging peacocks the island boasted an aviary, a farm, gardens, a number of fantasy castles, and a fountain powered by a nineteenth-century waterworks. What is more, it entailed travel through several wooded parks by *S-Bahn,* bus, and ferry. Brady had no desire to be with his mother outside of the privacy of the apartment, but I mobilized Ned for an expedition.

"Here, Ned. You be the photographer. You take pictures of the trip and then we'll send them to Dad." Ned happily assumed his role. He used more than half of the pictures on the trip, and took the rest within the first ten minutes of our setting foot on the island. As soon as the roll of film was gone, however, before we had explored, seen the birds, or picnicked, Ned was ready to go home. His arm was so painful walking any distance at all exhausted him. Distraction was not adequate to alleviate the pain. I had tested the "*Sei tapfer!*" and found it wanting. We wended our way back home where I read to him for the rest of the day. I was glad to go back to Dr. Schwalbach on Monday.

As I had expected, the gentle Dr. Schwalbach was concerned when I told the tale. He did not think it was right that Ned be in such pain a week and a half after the initial fall. He took a new set of X rays and poured over them. Again he found nothing. "It seems to be broken" he explained, "but I can't find anything on the X rays. I'll send them to a *Kollege* for another opinion. In the meantime we will treat it as if it is broken." He made a new splint and Ned was comfortable again. "Come back tomorrow," he said.

"Tomorrow" I returned willingly, but after Dr. Schwalbach unwrapped the splint, looked at the arm within, and wrote "*Kontrolle*" in Ned's record I was ready to be set free. When he said "Come back in two days," I balked. "Why do I need to come all the time?" I asked. "*Kontrolle*," he answered, in German. "What are we controlling for?" I persisted, irritated. "Bring him in on Friday," Dr. Schwalbach said firmly.

Sighing, I capitulated. Friday was a particularly difficult day for me. I was attending an international conference at the Max Planck Institute. I had really been looking forward to establishing and reestablishing contacts with scholars I had long known only through their work. Ghosts of my last year's preoccupation with Ned's problems threatened to shriek. But I tried to be reasonable about the whole thing. I knew that this was just a passing inconvenience, that Ned needed me, and that I would have other opportunities.

On Friday, I excused myself early to go to Dr. Schwalbach's. But I was not going to let things go on like this. As I traversed the city of Berlin on various *S-* and *U-Bahnen* I determined to face the doctor with my frustration. I wanted to know what the problem was, how the consulting *Kollege* had responded to the X rays the doctor had sent out. I wanted to move past this silly accident on a school playground and get back to a real life. I strode determined into Dr. Schwalbach's office.

He was not there. Instead his non-English speaking assistant greeted me and I lost my temper. "*Was ist das Problem?*" I fumed in my broken German. "What did the *Kollege* say? Why do we have to come here all the time? What is the problem with Ned's arm?" Chagrined and surprised, the poor man could do nothing. He knew nothing of the second set of X rays nor of the consulting *Kollege*. He was irrelevantly defensive about having removed Ned's splint the previous weekend, insisting that he was following instructions in Ned's record. I gave up and waited while he unwrapped Ned's splint, looked at the ever-less-swollen and painful arm, and wrote *"Kontrolle"* in Ned's record. I could only nod when he said to come back on Monday.

That evening I turned over and over in my mind possible explanations for Dr. Schwalbach's *Kontrollen*. "He just wants the money," one voice said. "Every time you visit and he writes '*Kontrolle*' in Ned's file, the insurance company pays him for an appointment." "He does not know what is going on," another opined. "He is worried and wants to stay on top of the situation." Or, less charitably, "He's clueless. He just wants to cover his back." The opinions crowded in from a host of people, most of whom I had met only in the previous month. The expatriot academic community in which I found myself was as dislocated as I. Nonetheless they offered their interpretations.

But the decisions about Ned's arm were mine to make. Even Rick was not much help. He had met Dr. Schwalbach, and was comfortable with what he had seen. Beyond that, though, we could not share the day-to-day experience of Ned's medical care. From afar he could only offer the wise constant that was reflected to me from all sides in my conversations with those who knew of Ned's medical past. "In any case, the arm is getting better. Relax, Joan," they all said. I said it too, again and again through the night as I lay sleepless and the bedside clock recorded another half hour gone by. "You've not yet put last year behind you; you are too quick to worry. Just relax!"

Genie and I tried to find ways to meet each other once a week. We tried lunches, but they were too disruptive to our days, so we switched to breakfast. This also was hard, both because we lived and worked in different parts of the city and because we had trouble identifying places open by eight o'clock. But we did not despair and every week tried a different experiment in early-morning dining—we'd meet at some tourist trap on the Kurfürstendamm, I'd bring rolls to her house, we'd stake out a dive halfway between our homes.

At the *Wissenschaftskolleg* I was beginning to make friends with Helge, a hard-driving young German philosopher of science. We were very different, as people and as scholars, but each was well equipped to understand the other's work. She did not have anything to offer about Ned's arm but she did have a son, Matteus, who was a promising friend for Ned. Although German, Matteus also was far from his home in Heidelberg. It was not easy for the two talkative children to play for sustained periods without language. Still, an hour here, an hour there was fun and they enjoyed each other.

At school Ned was also making friends. Every day seemed to bring a new announcement and accompanying enthusiasm: basketball, chess club . . . "Oh, Mom! Can I join Cub Scouts?" For this weekend the major activity was a "Run-a-thon," a five-mile run through the woods to benefit a South American orphanage. Ned would not have missed it for the world. "Will you sponsor me, Sean? . . . Great! And I'll sponsor you for five marks a kilometer [a mark was about 75 cents]."

"Where are you going to find twenty-five marks?" I asked after he had hung up.

"How about I vacuum the living room?"

Saturday morning we zipped through grocery shopping and then trekked across town so that Ned could run. The awkward splint did not bother him in the slightest as he loped along the wooded path. He beamed as he received a rubber band for each kilometer covered. *"Er ist so federnd!"* someone commented. "He is so feathered, so resilient." I let the easy poetry of the phrase sing to me as one after another of Ned's healthy friends crossed the finish line. The South American charity received more than fifty marks through Ned's efforts.

Monday Dr. Schwalbach was back. He reported that the consulting *Kollege* had found nothing in the X ray. My frustration began to dissipate as he removed the splint and Ned comfortably accepted an Ace bandage. Four days later, even that was pronounced optional. The arm was neither swollen, bruised, nor painful. I could not help thinking that in America the same results would probably have been achieved with two or three appointments and occasional telephone conversations, but at this point such speculations seemed unnecessary. The episode was soon to be water under the bridge; Schwalbach's attentive, gentle care had worked.

There was a problem, though: the elbow did not move. It was completely frozen in a right angle. "He's just afraid of the pain," Dr. Schwalbach explained, writing *"Kontrolle."* "He will move it in time, with the help of physical therapy." He wrote a referral form and indicated where we could find the physical therapist. He said nothing about ever coming back to see him. *"Er ist so jung,* he is so young," one of the nurses murmured as we went out.

The next week Ned and I got an appointment with the physical therapist. "It does not move," she explained unnecessarily. "There is nothing I can do now. Wait four weeks, and if it still does not move, come back. Or," she suggested brightly, "maybe you are in the States then! Maybe you go to your doctor there."

"No," I explained, "we are here for the year."

"Well, good-bye" she said.

"*Er ist so jung,*" clucked a sympathetic woman in the waiting room. As Ned and I walked out, his arm hung in a comfortable right angle at his side.

At home I struggled to balance my relief at the prospect of four weeks without a doctor's appointment with my growing conviction that all was not well. I certainly wanted no part of the clucking women who commented sympathetically on Ned's youth. He *was* young, certainly too young to be permanently disabled by a fall on a playground. I was quite clear about that, and willing to go to any lengths to insure that the current scenario did not have that outcome. But Dr. Schwalbach did not seem to think that there was any long-term problem, and in his immaculate office, with his gleaming X-ray machine and starched white coat he seemed the embodiment of aggressive, Western medicine. Yet the little boy he had sent home, apparently for the last time, seemed far from cured. I did not know how to respond to the passive waiting he and his physical therapist prescribed.

"This is Dr. Lyman. I am going to make an appointment for you to talk to Dr. Harlow."

"This is Dr. Gasparian. I have talked to Dr. Harlow, and he does not want to operate, but, I believe that the lesion is what is causing your son's seizures. I would like to present Ned's case to Dr. Bentley, who is a seizure surgeon from Yale."

"This is Dr. Gasparian. Dr. Bentley said he is not convinced that the lesion is a meningioma. But the surgeons seem to agree that it is in a tricky location, a bit deep, not easy to get. Dr. Weynolds suggested a stereotactic approach, essentially a needle biopsy. But others seemed to think that would be just as risky as an operation."

"This is Dr. Lyman. I've spoken to Dr. Gasparian and Dr. Bentley. I think we should send the pictures to Dr. Jennings at Boston Children's Hospital."

"This is Dr. Jennings. I have looked at Edward's pictures and I

*think it is too early to decide on anything. I think we should get
another set of pictures in three months and then we can do a
comparison."*

Ned's left elbow was a problem of a totally different order of magnitude
than a brain tumor. Nonetheless it struck me that Dr. Schwalbach
worked remarkably alone. Who reined him in if he was wrong? The
confusion, not to say chaos, of the process preceding Dr. Jennings's
advice did not lead to any clarity about what was taking place in Ned's
brain; somehow, though, it generated the assurance that was necessary
to sustain us through the wait. For the next several days, I pondered the
situation and observed my child.

Ned was his cheerful, active self; at times, in fact, his American
ebullience was a bit much for the more restrained denizens of the Villa
Walther. One weekend he invited Sean, a friend from school, to play,
and I gave them some sidewalk chalk. The outgoing fellow who had
unloaded it on me was German, so I had felt quite secure sending the
two boys into the sunny day to use it. Soon the Villa Walther's back patio
was gaily colored with maps of Europe and of America, with pictures of
Providence and of San Francisco, with flowers going up the pillars and
people standing on the ground. Satisfied with their efforts, the boys
signed off with flourishes and moved on to play by the *Seen.*

"What is *this*?" I heard the irate voices of a couple of sociologists
who had moved in downstairs. "Did your children do this?" they asked
of another fellow who was outside with his toddlers.

"No," he said. "My children aren't old enough to draw like this."

"But this is terrible! It has ruined our living place! It must not be
allowed!"

I cowered in the apartment, waiting for judgmental fingers to be
pointed at me and mine, but nothing happened. Late that night I crept
out with a bowl of water to erase the incriminating signatures. The rest
would just have to wait for the next rain; it was simply too much to handle with my little sponge. It was then that I first focused on the fact that
Berlin has very stable weather patterns; week after week passed, sunny
and dry. The sociologists just had to live with Ned's murals.

At school Ned was thriving. His no-nonsense teacher, Mrs. Harkin,
began making her mark; he began to take spelling seriously. In gym
class he qualified to be one of five fifth-grade boys to run in a citywide
competitive *"Waldlauf,"* a three-mile race through the woods. I signed
all the permission forms to release him from school on the nineteenth
of October.

Brady did not talk much about school but the signs were good. "I think I'll sign up to tutor mathematics. I've got plenty of time and they will pay me for it."

In my office I had begun again to work. The issue that was bothering me was the one that had arisen as I had tried to apply De Morgan's ideas to the Ned situation in the spring. It was clear to me that probabilistic thinking was simply silly as a model for the way we think in particular situations and that De Morgan knew it. That he had nonetheless spent ninety-seven pages writing about it could be attributed to simple mathematical exuberance, but I was not comfortable with this explanation. De Morgan was a thoughtful man who justified himself more carefully than that. I delved back into his probabilistic writing to look again at how he explained himself.

The answer I found had to do with De Morgan's views of how we know things. In a typically Victorian fashion, De Morgan saw Newtonian physics as the quintessential example of something successfully known. And like virtually all Victorian mathematicians, he saw knowledge as coming in two varieties that paralleled the essential distinction Newton had drawn between absolute and relative space.

Sometimes, we know things *necessarily, absolutely, certainly*. De Morgan would say this is how we know our own existence; it is also how we know basic mathematical truths like 2 + 2 = 4. Most things, however, we know only *contingently*, we have drawn them from our experience and cannot be absolutely certain that they are true. So, for example, we expect a December day to be cooler than an April day. We cannot be certain about it, though, and sometimes it is not the case.

When it comes to weather, it's obvious that we are uncertain in this way, but for De Morgan it was important to establish that almost everything we know, we know only contingently. For example, we may feel certain that the sun will rise tomorrow, but De Morgan would point out that it is not unimaginable that it wouldn't; it is possible to conceive of a world still dark at eight-thirty in the morning. So, for him, our knowledge that the sun will rise is not certain the way that mathematics is certain; it is not *necessarily* true.

The line between my certainty that the sun will rise tomorrow and my certainty that 2 plus 2 will equal 4 tomorrow can be difficult to draw, however. As I was trying to pin down the way De Morgan would explain it, I came across a letter he had written to his friend, William Whewell, who was a philosopher and the Master of Trinity College, Cambridge:

Camden Street, Oct. 21, 1846

My dear Sir [William Whewell],

. . .

I tried an experiment yesterday with my daughter of 8 1/3 years old as to the ideas of necessity, and there was a dialogue as follows:

A: If you let a stone go, what will happen?

a: It will fall, to be sure.

A: Always?

a: Always.

A: How do you know?

a: I'm sure of it.

A: How are you sure of it? Would it be true at the North Pole, where nobody has been?

a: Oh yes, people have been at the North Pole, else how could they know about the people who live there, and their kissing with their noses?

A: That's only *near* the North Pole. Nobody has ever been at the Pole.

a: Well, but there's the same ground there and the same air. Hotter or colder can't make the air heavier so as to make it keep up the stones. Besides I've read in the *Evenings at Home* that there is something in the ground which draws the stones. I am quite sure they would fall. Now, is there anything else you want to be a little more convinced of?

A: How many does 7 and 3 make?

a: Why, 10, to be sure.

A: At the North Pole as well as here?

a: Yes, of course.

A: Which are you most sure of, that the pebbles fall at the North Pole, or that 7 and 3 make 10?

a: I am quite as sure of both.

A. Can you imagine a pebble falling upwards?

a: No, it's impossible. Perhaps the birds might take them up in their beaks, but even then they wouldn't go up of themselves. They would be held up.

A: Well, but can't you think of their falling up?

a: Oh yes, I can fancy three thousand of them going up if you like, and talking to each other too, but it's an impossible thing, I know.

A: Can you imagine 7 and 3 making 12 at the pole?

a: (Decided hesitation.) No, I don't think I can. No, it can't be; there aren't enough.

Here her mother came into the room. As long as the questions were challenges from me it was all defiance and certainty, but the moment Mrs.

De M appeared she ran up to her and said, "What do you think Papa has been saying? He says the stones at the North Pole don't fall to the ground. Now isn't it *very* likely as they fall just as they do here and everywhere?" But she did not mention the 7 and 3 = 12 question, nor appeal to her mother about it.

As with so much else, I read this letter with new eyes in Berlin in early October. My mind wandered from the details of the distinction De Morgan wanted his daughter to understand, to the world of the child herself. It was reassuring to find concrete evidence that the reports of the demise of Alice's intelligence were premature, that at the age of eight she was still a perky character. But I was not completely mollified.

I was struck by the strangeness of the mold into which De Morgan was trying to fit his daughter's thinking. It was clear to me that the separation between the necessary and the contingent was not at all natural for the little girl. I felt creeping undertones of force in her father's insistence on finding it there.

My discomfort was fueled by worries about Ned. I was not confident that Dr. Schwalbach could see past his assumptions to see Ned's problem, any more than De Morgan could see past his views of truth to Alice's discomfort. But I was equally unsure that I could see past my own suppositions. In fact, if truth be told, I wasn't really sure what my suppositions were. I was uncomfortable but could not really justify it. So I tried to be patient, to wait and see.

I watched for signs that Ned's arm was loosening. There were none; he jumped, ran, climbed, and even rowed his boat, always with his left arm crooked like the wing of a chicken. The crisis arose over his clarinet. Ned's neighbor friend, Matteus, practiced his violin an hour every day and Ned was challenged to take up his instrument again. A few days after the physical therapist had sent us out, Ned triumphantly showed me that his arm was loose enough to maneuver the instrument to his mouth, albeit somewhat awkwardly. All his joy vanished, however, when he realized that his little and fourth fingers were not strong enough to push the keys.

As we discussed the situation it became clear that Ned felt little to nothing in these fingers and that the numbness extended up his forearm. This was not a result of fear. I called Dr. Schwalbach. His wife-receptionist told me, "Come tomorrow morning." When I protested that I wanted to consult over the phone, that he could call me when he was free, she firmly insisted that "Dr. Schwalbach is a very busy man. He does not do business over the phone. Come tomorrow morning."

The following morning, Ned joined Genie and me for breakfast by Dr. Schwalbach's office. We ate our rolls briskly and then went to confront the problem again, this time with Genie to act as translator and moral support. Squeezed with Genie, Ned, and me in the tiny examining room, Dr. Schwalbach listened carefully to my concerns. He gently cradled Ned's arm and moved his fingers. He asked Ned to make a fist, he pinched the little finger for a response. "He is fine," he assured us. "He is just afraid. He can feel the little finger when I pinch it. He can make a fist. There is nothing wrong." He let go of Ned's hand and the arm dropped easily to its crooked position at his side. The doctor smiled genially at Ned: "You must begin to move your arm," he instructed. "It won't hurt you." Ned promised to try.

Genie said that we wanted a second opinion; "Perhaps there is something wrong. Something that a specialist in elbows could see."

"I am a specialist," Dr. Schwalbach replied bluntly.

We wavered. "But if he has not gotten over his fear in the last couple of weeks, why should he get over it now?" I asked.

Dr. Schwalbach admitted that that was a question.

"We need a second opinion," Genie insisted.

Dr. Schwalbach wavered and then gave in. "All right," he said and arranged that after school Ned and I would go about a mile up the road to consult with a *Kollege*. Our intransigence had irritated him, but before we left he tried to heal the rift. "Come back in two weeks!" he said genially, and he shook my hand. I never saw him again.

Notfall (Emergency)

As he sent us off, Dr. Schwalbach had given us a note and three sets of X rays—the two he had taken while treating Ned and another he took just before we left his office. At the end of the school day Ned and I took the 110 bus up the Clayallee to the Otto-Hoffen-Heim. Clutching the large envelope, we got off the bus and contemplated the stucco hospital buildings that were our destination. I had resurrected the yellow spiral notebook for our appointments with Dr. Schwalbach, and I had carefully noted his instructions in it. We were to go to the *Kinderambulanz* or the *Kinderabteilung*, children's department, where we were to find "Waldemeyer." Dr. Schwalbach said that Dr. Waldemeyer might have time to see us if we caught him after his final operation of the day.

Ned and I slipped silently past the person controlling the entrance at the driveway to look at the large information board standing beyond his booth. For the *Kinderabteilung* it pointed down a road to the right of the *Hauptgebäude,* or main hospital building. We walked on, more doubtful with each step that took us beyond the sprawling hospital into a woods populated with a variety of small buildings including a trailer marked *Anästhesie*. A welcome informational board revealed that the *Kinderabteilung* lay ahead. We set off about fifty yards down a wooded path to a comparatively large, two-story outbuilding. The entrance hall had institutional seats to sit in; off of it were various corridors: those to the right were under construction, upstairs was Station H, straight ahead was *Gefasschirurgie,* to the left was a deserted corridor marked *Kinderabteilung*. Nowhere did the name Waldemeyer appear. Nowhere was there someone to consult.

"Oh, Mom! Can I have some cocoa?" Ned had focused on a machine dispensing hot drinks. I bought him some cocoa and myself a cup of coffee, and we sipped them together. Nothing happened except that the light began to fade. Another group came in and sat down and began to chat. A woman came from upstairs, bought herself a cup of coffee and went back up. A man came in with a child on crutches and they worked their way up the stairs. The workmen took a coffee break. The chatting group left. A family with many adults and one little girl came in and spoke to each other in Turkish. A woman with long blond hair came briskly down the path, her white medical robe flowing behind her.

"*Entschuldigen!* Excuse me!" I blurted. "Is this where I would wait to see Dr. Waldemeyer?"

"I guess so," she said. "He is in surgery right now. I don't know whether he will come back here or not." Buoyed by her admission that his presence in this place was not inconceivable Ned and I went back to our seats. The lights went on. We played three-dimensional tic-tac-toe on a pad on my knee.

Finally, about an hour after our arrival, I began to observe some movement in the corridor to the left. A secretarial messenger called the family with the little girl into one of its offices. I looked up expectantly, but doubted whether anyone could know we were there. I lurked in the corridor, finally plucking up the courage to knock on the closed door from which the messenger had emerged. In my fractured German I asked whether Dr. Waldemeyer was in.

"*Ja,*" I was told. "*Warten Sie, bitte!* Please wait."

"Does he know that we are here?" I persisted in German.

She responded in kind. "Who are you?"

I produced the X rays and the note from Dr. Schwalbach, which she put doubtfully on the desk. "*Warten Sie, bitte!*" she repeated. We went back to tic-tac-toe. The little girl and her family walked out of the corridor and into the night. A white-smocked man with wild hair poked his head into our room and scanned the people seated there. Apparently unable to find what he sought, he went back into the messenger's office and I followed.

"Are you Dr. Waldemeyer?" I asked in German.

"*Ja.*"

"Could we speak English?" I suggested, hopefully.

"Yes," he said, clearly a bit put out, "but who are you?"

I explained that Dr. Schwalbach had said to consult with him. "Oh, yes," he said briskly. "You have the X rays?"

I indicated the envelope on the desk. He picked it up and walked into an adjoining room. "Come!" he said.

Dr. Waldemeyer was about forty years old; his most unsurgeonly shock of hair frizzled around an energetic and cheerful face. He sat Ned on an examining table at the edge of a large room. A skeleton stood in one corner and various ancient corsets hung as somewhat macabre decorations high on the walls. Otherwise the room was empty and had the feeling of an elementary school lunchroom or gymnasium, cavernous and undelineated. The doctor leaned to look at Ned's crooked arm and tried in vain to budge it. He took out the three sets of X rays and put them on a lighted X-ray reader. He looked at them one after another. Ned slid off the table to stand at the doctor's elbow and look too. Dr. Waldemeyer bent over for a closer look. Ned followed suit. "That's it," the doctor said cheerfully, squinting with Ned at the most recent set. "See that?" and he pointed to a tiny fuzziness next to the bone of the upper arm. "Calcification!"

"You get an MRI," he went on, and faded to the phone in the next room. After a few calls he came back with a slip of paper. "Take this to X ray on Saturday," he said. "If she has time, Gretchen helps you then. When you have it, call me." I wrote the number of his answering machine in the yellow spiral notebook.

On the bus ride home Ned and I talked over our latest medical adventure. Ned was pleased by the novelty of the huge examining room, I by the easy assurance with which the surgeon proposed to open Ned's case to the wider world of the surrounding hospital. As for Dr. Waldemeyer, Ned thought he looked like a Brillo pad. I could see where he got his description but the doctor's hair was not all that I took away from the encounter. I had also noticed the man's hands, which were strikingly broad and strong. I had no trouble believing that Dr. Waldemeyer spent a good deal of his time setting bones.

The next morning I asked about the Otto-Hoffen-Heim at the *Kolleg*. Everyone I asked was clear that it was the premiere orthopedic hospital for Berlin and surrounding Brandenburg. What was more, the name Waldemeyer rang many bells. It was not hard to see that the man was the young scion of an old Berliner family with considerable medical connections. I was not sure I believed those who said that he was physician to the mayor of Berlin, but I could see that his name was well respected. In the walled town that Berlin had been, such things counted.

Still, in the evening, after Ned was safely stashed in his bed, I took advantage of the time difference to call Dr. Lyman. The novelty of a call from Germany achieved the previously impossible, an immediate connection: Over the 4,000 miles that separated us, I laid the case before Ned's American pediatrician. "It may be that there was some kind of break that has healed wrong," came the reassuringly familiar voice. "Or it may be that there is some kind of clot that is impeding motion. It sounds to me as if you're doing fine," he went on. "Let me know what Dr. Waldemeyer says after he has looked at the MRI."

For several hours over several days Ned and I pursued the MRI: we studied informational signs, huddled in waiting rooms, and tried to follow directions we at best half understood. The first plan failed. Gretchen was in charge of a small MRI machine, designed to take pictures of individual limbs. After a great deal of effort and pain it became clear that Ned's arm simply could not be straightened enough to fit into the tube. So, on Sunday night, I called Dr. Waldemeyer and left a message on his answering machine; he set the wheels in motion for Ned's elbow to be imaged in a full-body tube.

For Ned this performance was old hat. He looked over the tall, gangly Dr. Geisler as the man helped me fill out the German permission forms. "Dr. Geisler looks like a spaghetti man," he commented in the small cubicle where he was removing all metallic traces, including his jeans.

Underpants-clad on the machine's table, Ned showed off his knowledge to the doctor who was trying to figure out how to secure the small crooked arm with fixtures designed for adult straight ones. "You are going to take the pictures? In Rhode Island the nurses did this. Can I listen to music? You don't even have earphones? In Rhode Island they had earphones and I could listen to whatever radio station I wanted. They even let me bring my own tape. But then they erased it by mistake: they brought it by the machine. Since you are taking pictures of my elbow, can I swallow and open my eyes if I want?" Questions and comments fairly bubbled out of him as he was rolled into the tube. Dr. Geisler grinned, shaking his head in silent amazement as he retired to the glass booth.

I now knew enough about the technology to know that the doctor could see the images virtually immediately. I asked as we were leaving whether he could see any kind of problem. "I'm a radiologist, not an orthopedic surgeon," he said. "I do not know what Dr. Waldemeyer is looking for. I see fluid in the elbow, but you should not ask me."

Of course he was right, but I *had* asked him and was very comforted by the answer. Fluid in the elbow! It sounded like a piece of cake. I had been making mountains out of molehills all along. Fluid was just absorbed over time or could be drained with a syringe. My scenario for the future was comfortable. I called Dr. Waldemeyer's answering machine and he called back to say we should come in between nine-thirty and ten the next morning. I slept well.

The following morning Genie, Ned, and I had breakfast in the cafeteria of the hospital. She offered to stay for support, but I suspected the wait might be long and did not see any reason for her to hang around. So she went to work while Ned and I went to see Dr. Waldemeyer.

We settled into chairs and read a bit. Ned got a cup of cocoa from the hot drinks machine. I sent him out to run around the building.

Finally at about eleven-fifteen, the surgeon called us into his office. He took the MRI pictures and put them on his light box. "Oh!" he said immediately. "This is an emergency! He needs an operation right away."

Despite my shock I grinned at my son, for whom medical emergencies had entailed a mortal dimension. "It's no big deal," I said to Ned.

Taken aback at what appeared a contradiction, Dr. Waldemeyer insisted: "It is very serious. The *Ulnar Epicondyle* is completely broken off and is pushed into his elbow. We must operate right away."

"What does that mean?" I asked.

Dr. Waldemeyer explained, using his arm to identify relevant bones, that the *Ulnar Epicondyle* is part of the upper bone of the elbow; it can be felt as a spur with the *Ulnar Nerv*—the nerve that creates the "funny bone" effect—alongside of it. In an adult it is part of the bone; in a child it is cartilage, which explains why it did not show up on Dr. Schwalbach's X rays. Ned's had been knocked off in his fall, creating an *Abriss Fraktur* [explosive fracture]. It was, at the moment, jammed tightly into his elbow, creating the immobility that was so noticeable. It had to be taken out of the joint and refixed to the end of the bone where it belonged. The healing process was well on its way to making the current situation permanent, so an operation was essential.

"When will you operate?" I asked.

"We have to check the wards and the schedule of the operating theater," Dr. Waldemeyer replied. He made several phone calls and began to fill out forms.

"What about the *Waldlauf*? It's tomorrow," Ned said, tears in his eyes.

"I don't know," I replied. "We'll see."

"We go to the ward now," Dr. Waldemeyer said. "I operate tomorrow or the next day."

"Can't I just run tomorrow and then you operate on Friday?" Ned suggested hopefully.

"What?" Dr. Waldemeyer asked, his startled word sliding into the German "*Was?*" "No, of course not. This is very serious. We go to the ward now."

Ned and my autonomy vanished under the doctor's command.

"May I call my husband?" I asked.

"Of course!" he answered, "but first we go to the ward."

Dr. Waldemeyer led the way up the stairs, through some glass doors onto Station H. He strode past several rooms filled with beds and children, through another set of doors to a dimly lit corridor that sloped slightly upward. At the end of the corridor was another at right angles with several closed doors onto it. He opened one marked *Zimmer Acht* [Room Eight], and led us in.

Zimmer Acht was light and pleasant with large windows that opened onto a wooded area. Dr. Waldemeyer looked around happily, comfortably proud of the facilities in his hospital. "We usually put small children in here," he explained indicating the changing table. "But the ward is full and this is an emergency. In this room the mother spends the night," he went on indicating a couch along one wall. "That way she takes care of her child. We bring a bed for Ned."

When I asked how long we would be there, Dr. Waldemeyer replied with his special brand of authoritative cheer, "About ten days. Come, you call your husband." He took us into an office on the ward and dialed for an outside line. Then Ned dialed the Providence number: "Hello, Dad?" he said. Dr. Waldemeyer caught my eye, smiled, and left; I did not see him again until the operation was over.

Der Fuchs (The Fox)

In German, the letter *h* is pronounced as "ha," and Station H was an ironically appropriate designation for the situation in which Ned and I found ourselves. Our conversation with Rick was just moving past his sleepy shock at taking a phone call at six in the morning when a nurse opened the door to say in fiercely clipped English: "That is enough with the telephone." I ignored her and continued to explain the situation to Rick. Two minutes later she reappeared. "Stop the telephone!" she said. "I will in a minute," I replied, and went back to my explanation. Then Ned said a last good-bye to his father, and we emerged to face a firestorm. With a ferocity seemingly forged in equal measure by years of dealing with all-powerful doctors and non-German-speaking Americans, the nurse came for me. Her anger at our having used the ward's telephone to call the United States in the middle of the day poured out, on and on. The other nurses, who were all very young, gathered behind her to watch the show; they avoided eye contact as their leader berated me; Ned huddled under my arm. I passed from surprise through submission to an icy fury of my own.

"*Sprechen wir Deutsch!* Let's speak German," I commanded. "Perhaps you don't know how you sound in English." Stress improved both my vocabulary and my syntax. For the duration of our stay on Station H, my conversations with "Big Nurz," as she soon became known for lack of any other name, were in German.

This one moved on to administration. Various forms materialized around us and she explained in crisp bullets that we had better go first to *Anästhesie* [anesthesiology], since they closed at one, and then to register our presence in the *Aufnahme*, or registration office. Ned and I again set out to explore the wooded paths of the Otto-Hoffen-Heim. It took a couple of hours to negotiate the anesthesiologists' trailer and the paperwork of the *Aufnahme*. By two-thirty we were back in our quiet room on Station H, alone and hungry. I had checked out the hospital's only cafeteria as we passed it on our journey, but it closed at one-thirty.

"Is there something to eat?" I asked the young nurse I discovered down the hall and through the double doors.

"It is too late for lunch," the young woman quavered.

Big Nurz emerged to control the situation. "*Ach so,* you have come back," she fired. "There is food for the child outside of his room."

Ned and I investigated the cart parked outside his door and found a covered tray of tepid spaghetti with his name on it. We shared it happily. We sat in the quiet, pretty room. The large windows opened onto a small nature preserve, a *Naturschutzgebiet,* about two acres in size. The woods were pretty and a path ran through them. Station H was quiet and rather far away down the sloping corridor. We were alone. Ned tried the television but it did not work. I tried the telephone with the same result. The silence was palpable. We waited, almost afraid to speak. Nothing happened. I looked in the hall. It was deserted. I struggled with the various informational sheets trying to gain some insight into what we were to do. I managed to decipher the menu and times of meals. I learned that in this room the staff of Station H was happy to welcome parents and that, as a parent I was to cooperate with the support staff at all times. I found something that addressed the telephone but found it completely indecipherable. Ned fidgeted. We pored over the telephone materials complete with diagrams.

"Oh, I get it!" Ned jumped up and cheerily led the way past the nurses' station, through the ward, down the stairs to the room with the hot drinks machine. He pointed to another dispensing machine on the opposite wall. "You put twenty marks in there and then you get a thing to put in the phone!" I gave him a twenty-mark bill, which he fed into the machine with the mechanical ease of his generation. A small electronic chip came out. Triumphant, we took it past the bustling ward rooms, through the double doors to our silent room on the silent corridor.

We inserted it into the telephone. The television began to work and Ned settled back to cruise the German channels. The phone was my challenge. I pushed numbers at random. I dialed bravely as different signals flashed on the small screen. After about half an hour I figured out the right combination of moves to generate a dial tone. It took the same amount of time to actually reach someone.

Now the all-enveloping silence was pierced by the German of Ned's television, the noises of repeated dialing, and the English of my conversations. The latter began to produce results. Brady came over with nightclothes and Racky, Ned's ever-faithful stuffed animal. Other friends began to arrive with books and good cheer. We arranged a system whereby Brady would go from fellow to fellow for dinner and human contact; otherwise he was happy on his own in the apartment.

At seven o'clock visiting hours were over and everyone had to leave. Ned and I shared his dreary plate of cold cuts. Silence reigned and nothing happened. At seven-thirty a nurse instructed me to bathe Ned and cut his nails. She showed me where I could find sheets for my bed. We turned in early, ostensibly to rest before a busy day but in fact for lack of anything else to do. As we bedded down we were singularly clueless; the instruction to cut Ned's nails was as close as we came to an indication that Ned was, in fact, going to be operated on the next day.

The next morning both Ned and I were awake by seven. I was starving. I went down the corridor to check with a nurse because I did not want to be gone if Ned was going to be taken for the operation. It was a complicated subject to negotiate in the short, simple sentences of my German.

"Will my son be operated on today?" I asked.

"*Ja,*" she replied.

"At what time?" I went on.

"*Ich weiss es nicht,* I don't know," she answered.

"At eight o'clock, nine o'clock, ten o'clock, eleven o'clock?" I asked, looking for a ballpark figure.

"Perhaps," she answered.

"I want to eat," I tried.

"*Ja,*" she said. "But we do not have food for parents."

"I can go out."

"*Ja,*" she said.

Somehow we finally agreed that when I went out, Ned's bed could be wheeled to the relatively cheerful noise of the hall outside the nurses' station. I had a quick bite and came back. Ned was wheeled back to the room and we sat. Time passed. Some nurses came in and shaved Ned's arm.

"How long until the operation?" I tried.

"Perhaps an hour," they replied.

Fifteen minutes later the nurses returned with a sedative drink and prepared to take Ned for the operation. They covered his bed with a heavy blanket and wheeled him down the hall, down the elevator, and down the path to the main hospital building.

"What do you do when it rains?" I asked as we rattled along.

"*Eine Plane und ein Regenschirm,* a tarp and an umbrella." they replied simply. I grinned inwardly at the thought of transporting patients this way and wondered about snow and ice. I decided the question was above the level of my German.

We came to the main building. "*Sie können nicht hierhinein kommen*. You cannot come in here," they explained. The door closed behind them and the drowsy Ned.

Dr. Waldemeyer had said that the operation would be about half an hour, maybe an hour if there were complications. I added an hour on each side of that, for waiting, anesthesia, and recovery, and figured that Ned would be out in about three hours. It was a quarter to ten. I retrieved my book from the silent room and went for a cup of coffee in the small cafeteria. It was basically deserted, but I took comfort from the occasional human presence as I determinedly read. By noon, when people started to come for lunch and nonmedical people were no longer welcome, two-and-a-half hours had passed since I had seen Ned. I returned hopefully to Station H, but he was not there.

At one o'clock he was still not there. "Do you know when my son will come back?" I asked one of the young nurses.

"*Ich weiss es nicht*, I don't know" she answered and went on with her business.

Restless, I wandered towards the hot drinks machine. I paused on the way down the stairs to look outside. In the grassy area behind the building lay a fox soaking up the warmth of a patch of sun. She was curled in a loose ball, with her tail over her nose. I watched. A sleeping animal does not provide much action, but I could see her breathe. Time passed and as the sun moved inexorably along, the shadow of Station H began to eclipse the fox's warm patch. As the sun receded from her back, she opened her eyes. Slowly she uncurled her tail, and laid it, gleaming red, in the sun. She got up and stretched luxuriously. There was nothing crafty or sly in her as, looking neither to the right nor the left, she calmly trotted into the woods of the *Naturschutzgebiet*.

She came to me as an omen of health. My anxiety over Ned was replaced by an equally intense desire to tell what I had seen. I returned to Station H and searched out an animal poster of the kind people put in children's wards in an attempt to make them less grim. I found one in the dim corridor leading to Ned's room, which had a fox peeking out from around a tree. As I stood there contemplating my next move, Big Nurz materialized at my side.

"What is this called in German?" I asked, pointing at the little figure.

"Ein Fuchs," she responded.

"I just saw a fox!" I said proudly.

"Ach so!" she said happily and she opened up. She told me that there were several foxes that lived in the woods around the hospital. They had appeared unexpectedly when the wall came down; the grim structure had not only kept East German people from the city but East German wildlife as well. Now, in the spring the fox mothers would bring their young frolicking around the outbuildings; the children loved watching them. Big Nurz delighted in them as well. Telling about the foxes she became warm and calm.

I plucked up my courage to ask about Ned whom I now had not seen for more than four hours. *"Ich weiss es nicht,* I don't know," came the accustomed response, but more came as well. Big Nurz told me to go for a walk in the woods; that I was not needed on the ward at the moment. It did not matter whether I was there the instant he returned from the operation because he would be sleepy anyway. I would be needed later. Now I should go out and take care of myself in the crisp autumn afternoon.

Grateful to tears for her responsiveness I took her advice. I spent the next hour wandering the woods. I knew that somewhere near the fox was sleeping in the underbrush; I knew that somewhere near people were taking good care of Ned.

Ned was wheeled back to the room on Station H between three and three-thirty, more than five-and-a-half hours after he had been wheeled away. His arm was engulfed in a huge plaster cast, from which protruded a small tube ending in a vile plastic bag of slowly draining blood. He was pale, groggy, and, for the most part, sweetly asleep; however he became reassuringly grumpy as various anonymous medical personnel asked him what he could feel and commanded him to move his fingers. After about half an hour a new personage appeared and began to preside over the project of wheeling Ned away again. I followed, not understanding the issue, but unwilling to let Ned out of my sight.

Our destination was the large *Gipsraum,* the room where casts were made and adjusted. There a young medic struggled with the project of slitting Ned's cast to allow for swelling. Others hung in the background or walked around the room. I recognized that the saw could not cut Ned, but it made me feel sick to watch people clumsily sawing and pawing his limp arm, while the bag of blood bobbled from it. I headed for the door. Dr. Waldemeyer opened it before I got there. Buoyed by his presence, and by his English, I returned to Ned's side.

Dr. Waldemeyer took over with the saw and deftly pried the two sides of the cast apart. At least when he was at the helm there was nothing to the procedure, and he expounded on the operation as he performed it. He fairly vibrated with triumph as he related how the *Ulnar Epicondyle* had taken the *Ulnar Nerv* with it as it lodged itself in the joint. "Dr. Dannehl," apparently a consulting neurosurgeon, "said he has seen it only twice in twenty-five years and both times there was no feeling and no movement in the hand!" he crowed. Dr. Waldemeyer looked admiringly at Ned, or rather at his plaster-encased elbow. "It is all right, now," he went on. "We put in two pins for the bone and put the nerve back." He turned to his disciples: "He can move his fingers, *ja?*" and fairly bounced in his tennis shoes at the positive response. This was a man who loved bones, joints, and muscles. The current focus of his interest was my son's elbow, and his joy in it was irresistible.

When I returned from the *Gipsraum,* I found Genie in tears because Big Nurz had exploded when she asked for a vase. Dr. Waldemeyer's enthusiasm did not carry him far enough to see Ned for more than a few minutes in the four additional days he kept us on Station H. Ned sat cheerfully in bed, his left arm hidden in a mass of plaster. In terms of the hospital regime, very little happened; Friday, Saturday, and Sunday crept by with no rhyme, reason, or action that I could make out.

At the *Wissenschaftskolleg* the new year was officially beginning. Thursday, the day of Ned's operation, all new fellows' went with the administration on a boat trip though Berlin's canals. Friday I had been invited to a dinner party at Helge's to meet some of Berlin's physicists and historians of science. "Brady, will you come and take your mother's place?" I told myself firmly that missing an evening was not important; Ned would soon be out of the hospital, the problem with his arm a faint memory.

On Saturday Rick was coming, at least we hoped he was. He had been unable to reach us at the tenuous telephone in our room and Big Nurz had effectively cut off all communication in the other direction. Genie relayed the message that he was desperate and flying in for a lightening visit to check on Ned. Brady went to the airport to try to meet him. There were several flights to choose from, though, and after he did not find Rick on three of them, Brady and I agreed it was time for him to give up the wait and come to the hospital. Rick knew where we were and could find us by himself.

About an hour after Brady and I hung up the phone, my lanky son arrived to flop on the couch.

"How was dinner at Helge's?"

"It was fine. I wore my blazer. Was that right?"

"Yup. I bet you looked great."

"We had fish with bones, and I ate it. I tried to help with clearing the table and stuff. Mostly they talked German, but I did my best."

"It sounds as if you were a trouper."

The door flew open. "*Keine Bewegung!*" Rick commanded.

"Oh, Dad!" Ned squealed.

"Dad, you are so silly!" Brady said suavely.

"Hush," I laughed. "The nurses will have a fit!"

Soon thereafter Dr. Waldemeyer arrived to smile, shake Rick's hand, and ask Ned how he was. He nodded appreciatively at the positive answer and left. It was a brief but positive contact; Rick liked him.

Completely jet-lagged, Rick could not sustain the energy of his entrance for long. Soon he displaced Brady on the couch and we moved into a desultory afternoon. At some point some nurses and a doctor came to take out Ned's blood bag.

"*Husten!*" they told him. "Cough!" He did and they yanked and that was the end of that. It was the only medical action in the entire weekend.

Rick stayed the night with Ned, which freed me to leave with Brady. We walked to an *Imbiss,* a hot dog stand, on the corner and each ordered a *halbes Hähnchen,* half chicken, to go. We cradled the foil-wrapped bundles in companionable peace as the 110 bus carried us home.

"Mom. I forgot to tell you. I let the bath run too long on Thursday and it overflowed into the hall."

"What did you do about it?"

"Well, I vacuumed the carpet, put towels on it, and walked on them. Then I put new ones down and walked on them. Then I opened all the windows for a while. It's dry now."

"Sounds good, sweetie. What did you do with the towels?"

"I was going to wash them but I haven't had time."

After we had supped, I commandeered the least dirty towel and sank blissfully into my first bath in four days. Then Brady and I did laundry.

On Sunday Rick and I left Brady with Ned and stole the afternoon together. About a block from the apartment we met the sociologists who were intently discussing the electoral policies of the European Union. We blandly accompanied them to the Villa Walther. Ned's artwork sparkled in the afternoon sunlight.

They disappeared into their first-floor apartment. Rick and I laughed guiltily as we climbed the stairs to ours. "I wish it would rain!"

Sunday night was Rick's night with Brady, and I returned to *Zimmer Acht*. If we could get Ned home on Monday, the family could have a whole day together before Rick flew back to Providence on Wednesday.

By Monday morning Ned had been sitting in the hospital more than twice as long as he had been for his neurosurgery. His cast was heavy and unwieldy, but it did not seem sufficient to keep him bedridden indefinitely. We were contemplating a recreational walk through the *Naturschutzgebiet* when we were stopped by a determined nurse who said "*Die Ärzte kommen*, the doctors are coming." We retreated to the room and were soon visited by three unmistakable *Ärzte*. One was about sixty; the other two were unfamiliar, young, and very respectful. They ranged themselves at the end of Ned's bed and stared at him.

Our German evaporated. It did not much matter because they were not interested in talking to us. A younger doctor explained the case to the older man. He listened and regarded Ned gravely. When he realized that six weeks had passed between the time that Ned fell and the time of his operation, he was appalled.

"You let this go by for six weeks?" he asked me in amazed German.

I scrambled to explain, but he was not interested in my broken German tale of a doctor gone wrong. He was neither the first nor the last of the doctors I spoke with to emphasize the crucial importance of early treatment for elbows. He was neither the first nor the last to look balefully at me when he realized so much time had elapsed between the fall and the operation. But as far as I can tell, neither he nor any of the others with whom I spoke ever made any move to communicate their displeasure to Dr. Schwalbach. The responsibility for identifying and avoiding poor medical care was simply mine, and I had failed utterly. The passivity these doctors enforced on Rick and me by their incoherent mutterings at our son's bedside rankled all the more as I mulled over this attribution of guilt. Not that it mattered. The important doctor and his followers left without a backward glance.

Soon thereafter we did the same. Our next query to the powers at the nurses' station revealed there was no more reason for us to stay. Eagerly we packed up all of our belongings, put the parental bedding in the dirty-clothes hamper, and forgot our snack food in the small refrigerator. As we walked out carrying our assorted clothes and books, Big Nurz was fiercely establishing her dominance over a new young doctor on the ward. We, on the other hand, were home free to go home, and there we luxuriated in a full day of time. On Wednesday, Rick flew back to Providence and Ned went back to school.

A couple of days later Dr. Schwalbach called me up. Apparently he had received the effusively polite form letter I had seen in Ned's file, informing him of Ned's diagnosis and progress.

"How is Ned doing?" he asked.

"He is fine," I answered. "At least for the moment. It is hard to tell how his arm is with the cast on."

He agreed. "I'm sure it is fine, now. He is young. He heals well."

"I hope so," I said.

There was a pause. "I did not see the problem," he said. "I really looked, you know. It was just too small. I could not see it."

It was just too small. I could not see it.

Dr. Schwalbach's X-ray machine enabled him to see sharp images of the bones that lay hidden deep within Ned's arm, but it did not give him insight. The X ray was clear but it was also clear, in our fifteen appointments spread over more than five weeks, that Ned's arm did not move. Over and over again Dr. Schwalbach and his *Kollege* had denied the reality of what they could not see.

Sei tapfer.

He is just afraid to move it.

Villa Walther

The Villa Walther was filling up. We had come two months early to accommodate the boys' school schedule and in September we had shared the large building only with Matteus's family and the sociologists. However, by October 23, when Ned came home from the hospital, all of its approximately twenty apartments were inhabited by various fellow-families. They hailed from all over the world, which meant that in addition to the usual challenges of introductions we had to negotiate language. A Chinese man and I heroically conversed for half an hour in German before he realized I was American and settled comfortably into the English he had learned in a twelve-year career in Colorado. My next-door neighbor just giggled in despair when I tried to strike up a German conversation, and she laughed even harder at attempts in English. After several brief and hilarious interchanges we finally realized that our common language was French. When I heard another colleague from Lebanon conversing easily with her I assumed French was the right approach there as well. But when I introduced myself with my most polished "*Je m'appelle Joan Richards. Et vous?* My name is Joan Richards. And yours?" the Middle Eastern specialist just laughed.

"I'm as American as you are," she said. "Can't we just speak English?"

The Russians spoke French. The Africans spoke French. The French spoke French. Some of the northern Europeans seemed able to deal with almost anything: English, French, German, Italian, Spanish, Arabic, Japanese. The Italian spoke German. The English spoke English with a wonderful array of accents and dialects.

For the Richardses, the apex of the English speakers were the Wests, Christopher and Beth, who moved with their three-year-old twins into the large apartment off Ned's decorated terrace. Christopher was interested in the social philosophy of accounting, the ways that accounting practice affects the shape of the society that embraces it. Beth was a doctor, who had taken a year off to accompany Christopher to Berlin. At all hours of the day, their three-year-old twins, William and

James, could be heard piping out the most wonderfully clipped English in their chirrupy little voices.

There was humor in the architectural extravagances of the Villa Walther; the *Kolleg*, where we worked, was simply elegant. Large beautiful halls, polished curving stairways, beautifully proportioned public rooms and, where you entered, a magnificent fresh flower arrangement, five or six feet high. Purple, red, yellow; sinuous, massive, exuberant, every week the flowers were different, every week they were lovely. The seminar room was in the back, frighteningly formal with floor-to-ceiling windows and external stairs that swooped to the landscaped lawn and yet another *See* beyond.

Where the Max Planck Institute exuded scruffy sincerity, the *Wissenschaftskolleg* exuded polish. Its finish was maintained by a staff, which was as numerous as the fellows, and which ranged from cooks and janitors through computer specialists, librarians, and secretaries to the heights of administration. Most of them were fluent in English and German, many spoke French as well; those who held professional positions routinely attended seminars. The *Verwaltung*, the administration, was a real presence at the *Kolleg*, permanent where the fellows were not.

Very visible among the fellows were a number of elder academic statesmen: former college presidents, directors of foundations, retired academic nobility. With them were others like Christopher or me; middle-level academics working to make our way. And then there were those less established yet: Germans working for their *Habilitation*—somewhere between American postdoctorates and professors. The positions were clear and unquestionable. We all knew our places, and were all working hard to maintain or better them.

Downstairs was the dining room, where, every weekday, the fellows supped. Lunches were superb, formal, and not to be taken lightly. After the first seminar I was blissfully satisfied with my bowl of cream of mushroom soup only to be surprised by another course: potatoes, broccoli, and a full trout. I picked at the offerings while I listened to the German man at my left who was discussing the layout of Berlin and bemoaning the hasty nineteen-fifties architecture of the reconstructed west.

The waitress cleared the plates around me. Finally she could avoid the issue no longer. "*Schmeckt's nicht?* Don't you like it?" she asked concerned.

"*Doch! Es schmeckt! Aber ich habe genug gegessen.* On the contrary! It's delicious. But I've had enough."

Horrified, she fetched her superior. We went through the issue again, but my explanation was simply incomprehensible. Finally they realized the problem. *"Ach so! Sie ist Amerikanerin!* She is an American! It makes Americans squeamish to eat fish when the head and the tail are still attached." So, whenever they served trout in the future mine came without the head and the tail. I realized I had better eat.

We had lunch four days a week: on Thursdays it was dinner. Spouses were allowed, children were to dine elsewhere. Wine flowed freely and conversation could be sparkling.

At the first of the Thursday dinners, I sat at a table with Bill McAllister, recently retired after a stellar career first as the provost of a major Midwestern university then as a centrally important federal science advisor. He was sitting with the rector [director] of the *Wissenschaftskolleg*. It was language that drew me there; I knew Bill did not speak German and that no one would ask him to. Jane, Bill's wife, was also there; as high powered as he, she was just about to go to Sweden to pick up the Nobel prize on behalf of Pugwash, the scientific antiwar group with which she had worked from the early nineteen-fifties.

My role at the table was to listen, and I did as the two men discussed the state of German academics after the dismantling of the wall, and the intellectual situation in America with Newt Gingrich, who was then at his most powerful.

After the men had talked for a bit, the rector turned graciously to Jane: "I hope you are enjoying your apartment in the Villa Walther."

"Yes," Jane replied. "It's fine. But don't Germans have double beds? Ours is just two single beds side by side. And we each have a separate comforter. How do Germans get together?"

"Get together?" The rector, looked aghast at the seventy-five-year-old woman at his right.

"Yes," Jane went on unperturbed. "Bill and I like to sleep together, we like to touch each other. Surely Germans must do that too! But how do you get together from two separate beds?"

I listened gleefully as the German man and American woman tried to figure out the limits of public and private at *Wissenschaftskolleg* dinners. Ultimately Jane's American straightforwardness routed the polished rector, who brusquely closed the conversation: "You'll have to talk to Frau Schultz if you have trouble with the bedding. She is in charge of the apartments."

Thursday nights were adult affairs—except for the first Thursday of every month. This was children's night. Children's night was a wonderful and much anticipated event. A table was lavishly laid in one corner of the fellows' dining room. Coca-Cola and candy were provided in endless supply—as far as I could tell, very little else was consumed. Many fellows were childless, had grown children, or had left their families at home when they came to Berlin. Still, there were about ten children, the overwhelming preponderance of whom were male, between the ages of ten and fourteen. At almost sixteen Brady was the eldest, and at six feet, three inches, the largest; he led the unruly polyglot pack through Ping-Pong tournaments and rambunctious games of manhunt in the darkened halls of the *Kolleg*.

Ned with his cast, plunged cheerily into the action, unabashed by the linguistic variety around him. He also looked out for the little twins, with whom he was joined by language and who were the first people ever to regard him as a source of wisdom and stability. He reveled in the grown-up role. Several times during an evening he would shepherd the little boys to their receiving parents: "William fell and bumped his knee," or "James says he's scared in the dark room upstairs."

For two hours a week the *Kolleg* offered German classes to foreign fellows. They were taught at three levels. *Gruppe A* was heroic in its challenge, which began with polite greetings. *Gruppe C* was heroic in accomplishment, and spent two hours every Wednesday afternoon heatedly discussing the week's seminar in German. *Gruppe B* was heroic in little but its doggedness. Comprised of all the poorly defined incompetents between *A* and *C*, we met behind closed doors in the hour before the seminar, so our teacher could help us to understand the precirculated abstracts. We did not have much more to lose in terms of prestige.

We learned a lot of German in *Gruppe B*, but except for quiet improvement in passive understanding, our increasing proficiency was not noticeable in the *Kolleg*. We were surrounded by German speakers, but their facility with English was daunting. In the rare moments that we of *Gruppe B* tried to speak German, we would be smoothly rescued at the first sign of confusion. This meant we rarely got past the first sentence before the conversation would switch to English.

The stalwart exception was the receptionist, Frau Breunig, who reigned in a little office to the right of the elegant flower arrangements. Frau Bruenig's English was just fine, but she would soldier through with us in German. Grandmama would have loved the way she took charge, looked you straight in the eye, and enunciated carefully. Taken in by her no-nonsense clarity, one fumbling fellow after another forgot to be self-conscious and entered the conversation. Frau Breunig was a great support, and I looked forward to our daily German chats as I picked up my mail by her desk.

By now, my photocopies and microfilms from Cambridge had arrived and I had turned my attention from De Morgan to his somewhat younger compatriot, Robert Leslie Ellis, who published two important papers on probability theory in the middle of the century. I found Ellis's first paper interesting because he seemed to see what my experiences with Ned's doctors had led me to believe, that it was utterly false to think about human decision making in terms of rational calculation. De Morgan had acknowledged that when one had a deep personal, emotional stake in a situation, probability calculations were not adequate to model how one thinks, but for Ellis this was not enough. The younger man insisted that De Morgan's probabilistic way of thinking was not adequate to any real situations.

Consider the simple example of a person sitting on a riverbank watching boats go by. If ten boats go by, each flying a flag, what is the probability that the next boat will fly a flag? "Let us suppose the ten vessels [which flew flags] be Indiamen," Ellis objected. "Is the passing up of any vessel from a wherry to a man of war, to be considered as constituting a 'next occasion'? or will an Indiaman only satisfy the conditions of the question?" So, whereas De Morgan thought one could crisply calculate the probability that the next ship would fly a flag, Ellis saw that such a calculation would not be crisp at all. He insisted on the reality of what I had found as I tried to rationally calculate the probability of Ned's seizures, that in real examples the attempt to mathematize rational thinking was hopelessly inadequate.

Ellis's work would be an important part of my book and I wanted to understand his position better. I could start at the beginning, because from the time he was ten Ellis kept a diary. It was not a particularly fun read. One of my more dubious honors is to have been elected the "most serious girl" in my senior class in high school, but even I never closed my diary entries with a judgment of whether I had spent the day well or not. From the age of twelve Ellis did.

By the time he was sixteen the heaviness was almost unbearable. When he wasn't recording how many pages of mathematics he had read, Ellis was finding ultimate meanings. So, for example, after a social morning in town, he came home alone "—like many a man who goes to his long home—after losing all the sets of companions he was with in life."

In the late eighteen-thirties, when De Morgan was cleanly dividing his life between the domestic unknown and the calculated building of career, Ellis was attending Cambridge. In 1838 he finished first in his class in mathematics. This triumph was not enough to brighten his mood, though. On the contrary, the exhaustion of the effort left him in a state of physical and emotional collapse. Everything he did thereafter was presented with ultimate overtones. In 1848 he planned a trip to the Continent for his health: "I am not sorry to draw off from Cambridge before the final separation comes."

By the time I came across this interpretation I was thoroughly exasperated, but at this point Ellis's gloom began to be borne out by his experience. On his trip he became desperately ill with rheumatic fever. After three months, he recovered enough to get out of bed but not much more. "I am much bent forward and the head a good deal down on the chest and immovable sideways or nearly so. I drag one foot in walking partly from the knee and partly from general weakness. My hair is somewhat thin and eye very hollow and half inflamed. Altogether I am excessively repulsive to myself—as I have long been more or less. It is curious when at the end of the day's journey I am extracted from the carriage to see how the people look at me—not that I see half of them, though I pull my hat off as a mark of respect to the master or mistress of the house of whom I see at first only the skirts or gaiters etc." This seemed horribly real; I cringed as I read.

Ellis never recovered from his European tour. He became so gloomy that he could almost joke about it: "Today the dog died. I find that neither flowers nor the thought of their withering cheers me." His limbs became ever more twisted with arthritis, Bright's disease caused his eyes to bleed, his heart beat irregularly. He wrote poetry that his sister circulated among her friends.

The flower was crooked in the bud
It was a sickly faded flower
What seeks it now? however fair
It still had died before this hour.

He worked mathematics problems to pass the time. De Morgan sent him the four-color problem, but he did not take it up. Death became an ever-more-present preoccupation. "I write to ask you not to come tomorrow. I do it with the more regret as I cannot but think it doubtful whether I shall ever see you again." The message beat a numbing refrain through the final ten years of Ellis's correspondence. "The curse of Moses 'Thy life shall hang in doubt before thee and thou shalt fear day and night and have none assurance of thy life' has been fulfilled here if ever anywhere—" Ellis wrote to a friend about a month before he died. This seemed a real cri de coeur and it made me uncomfortable. It called to mind De Morgan's hypothetical man contemplating death before an urn with an unknown ratio of black to white balls. Ellis seemed to have made a similar connection. Even as he was collapsing, his legs crumpling, his eyesight fading, he wrote a second probability paper attacking De Morgan's interpretation.

Here Ellis tried again to explain that in real life there is no distinction between the person contemplating a situation and the situation itself, that the boundary between the knowing person and things that are known is artificial. "Man in relation to the universe is not *spectator ab extra* [observer from outside], but in some sort a part of that which he contemplates," Ellis insisted from within his twisted body. We do not sit outside of life's possibilities like entrants in a raffle. We do not calculate the odds as we make decisions about our future. Life's possibilities are us and we them; we are in their midst at all times. "The thoughts we think are, it is true, ours, but so far as they are not mere error and confusion, so far as they have anything of truth and soundness, they are something and much more. The *veritas essendi* [essential truth] . . . is the fountain from whence the *veritas cognoscendi* [known truth] is derived. . . . Only on the horizon of our mental prospect earth and sky, the fact and the idea, are seen to meet, though in reality the atmosphere is everywhere present. Everywhere it surrounds and interpenetrates the [black earth] on which we stand—making it put forth and sustain all the numberless forms of organization and of life."

When I began reading Ellis I had found it hard to agree with Sophia De Morgan, who wrote that he gave her "the impression of an almost perfect moral nature." I found his diary dreary, his correspondence self-absorbed, his poetry insipid. In his second paper on probabilities, though, I caught a glimpse of what had so inspired her. For Ellis mathematics was not a flight to a pure, absolute realm of thought, separate from the common and the relative. The truths that could seem so far away, "on the horizon of our mental prospect," were in fact all around: "the atmosphere is everywhere present." Ellis breathed this truth in his darkened room, it blew around his wheelchair in the garden. Everywhere it surrounded and interpenetrated the black earth on which he lived although he could no longer stand. As I breathed the atmosphere in my office in Berlin, I was transfixed by the immediacy of Ellis's vision.

* * *

Reading Ellis was absorbing and wrenching, and it was often a great relief to put it down for the *Kolleg's* series of weekly colloquia. Many of the presentations were in German and stretched my comprehension to its limits and beyond. The subjects were as diverse as the fellows: in the first weeks I learned about city planning in Berlin, Japanese sociology, and the structure of the flu virus.

Another week, a biologist presented his work on microscopic colonial organisms.

"Colonies of this kind, type A, can reproduce themselves even if only a single cell remains. When the feedback systems with the neighboring cells are interrupted they compensate and begin to reproduce by fission. . . ."

"There might be a few cells left, close to the Labe vein. I did not want to scrape it down too hard."

"When one is dealing with type B colonies things are much more precarious. These feedback systems are essential to the health of each of the cells, and if they are interrupted, the cells will die. With this kind of system reproduction is by budding, not by fission—unless the whole structure is intact, they cannot reproduce. The advantages of this kind of system . . ."

"This kind doesn't come back."

Just when I had felt myself secure, in control, and safe my mind hurled me into uncertainty. "Man in relation to the universe is not *spectator ab extra* [observer from outside], but in some sort a part of that which he contemplates," Ellis reminded me. I willed myself to sit quietly through the rest of the technical talk but was unable to meet my goal of one intelligent question at the end.

Genie and I continued our weekly breakfasts all over town. On many evenings new and old friends would come for dinner and a visit. Clare swooped in, all chic and English, and fascinated the boys with her voice and vocabulary. Liza appeared in a Tibetan hat trimmed with fox fur; she had a way of taking Ned absolutely seriously that was a delight to him. Plato traded mathematical challenges with Brady. From just down the hall, Helge dropped in for an occasional glass of wine and intense conversation. I began to feel connected in Berlin.

✩ ✩ ✩

Brady was becoming ever more enmeshed in school.

"Will you pick up eggs, milk, and pasta on your way home today, Brady?"

"I don't know whether I'll be home before the stores close, Mom. I'm tutoring Tina today, and she's really in trouble. I don't see how she got this far in math! I'm not sure she knows what the trig functions are. She can't even factor binomials!"

"Well, don't overwhelm her. Just work on one *or* the other."

"I know. I thought we'd work on binomials today and do the trig stuff next week. Bye!"

Weekends continued to be a challenge for Ned and me. Brady just retired to his room, but Ned needed action. His school friends lived far away and his casted arm eliminated all of the sporting activities, like swimming, I'd projected for him. So, we went on a series of exploratory expeditions.

One Sunday we took a long *U-Bahn* ride to the Spandau Zitadel, a fifteenth-century fort. We walked along the walls that jutted, star-shaped, into the waters of the Havel. We contemplated its long and complex history of warfare, most recently as a storage place for Nazi nerve gas, and then visited the arts colony it currently houses. There were weavers and candle makers. A potter identified us as Americans and tried, without success, to remember the capital of Rhode Island. We bought a candle that played "Happy Birthday" for Brady, whose birthday was coming up. We then went to the other side of the court-yard to visit the remnants of the oldest Jewish cemetery in Berlin.

Another week we visited the Charlottenburg Schloss, the palace Friedrich I built for Sophia Charlotte. It was here that Leibniz had worked, and Caroline had grown up, but I found Sophia Charlotte intriguing in her own right. She died when she was only thirty-seven of a cancer in her throat. "Do not pity me," she said to a lady-in-waiting who was weeping at her bedside. "I am at last going to satisfy my curios-ity about the origin of things, which even Leibniz could never explain to me, to understand space, infinity, being and nothingness; and as for the King, my husband—well I shall afford him the opportunity of giving me a magnificent funeral, and displaying all the pomp he loves so much." When Ned and I got there, we found that the gargantuan castle breathed Friedrich's spirit more than that of his wife, though. Ned did not want to go in, so instead we walked around in the gardens deciding what we would plant if we were in charge.

A favorite destination was the Grunewald See—a lake about three-quarters of a mile from the Villa Walther. As its name suggests, the lake was in the Grunewald, a large wooded park that for decades had provided walled, now unwalled, Berlin with hundreds of acres of wooded space. Most of the forest is about fifty years old, because the previous one was cut down for fuel in the immediate postwar period. The replanted parts are at times laughably regular, criss-crossed by absolutely straight paths. Nonetheless, the wood was lovely and it was a boon to find it less than a mile from our house.

On Saturdays and Sundays, whatever the weather, the paths around the Grunewald See were full of Berliners with their dogs: big dogs, well-behaved dogs. German shepherds cavorted around their family groups. Rotweilers and great danes swam from the designated *Hundbadstelle* [dog bathing place], splashing, barking, swimming after sticks. They trotted with their owners, often in twos or threes, down paths through the woods. They milled around the trailer *Imbiss* where Ned and I bought *Rostbratwurst* for lunch. *"Komm, Max!"* and Max would come.

Near the *Imbiss,* was the Grunewald Schloss, a sixteenth-century hunting lodge. Ned and I wandered through its open gates while eating ice cream bars. Inside it was still. Grass grew soft between the stones of the enclosed courtyard. On the right were the stables, on the left the main lodge building of clean, yellow stucco. In the surrounding walls were numerous doors and windows; habitations for stableboys and other servitors. The *Schloss* gave me a new view of the major streets I'd been traveling in Berlin. The Kurfürstendamm became the street of the *Kurfürsten*, the electors. It was the route they took to the Koenigsallee, the King's street, which led to the hunt in the Grunewald.

It required a powerful act of the imagination to see the *Kurfürsten* traveling the twentieth-century streets, but in the inner space of the castle's courtyard I could feel their presence. Ned and I went into the small art museum housed in the castle, and there we could see the *Kurfürsten* and their world in paint. Centuries melted and melded in views through the windows of the little *Schloss*. The sky was blue, the autumn air was crisp. Grasses grew down to the glittering water; across it grew the trees. There were foxes in the woods and, if people were to be believed, wild boar as well. The twentieth-century world of Sunday strollers and leashed dogs was nowhere to be seen or heard.

"This place is cool," Ned said as he contemplated a sixteenth-century picture of a two-headed calf.

11/4/95

Dear Rick,

Well, I think Berlin beat Providence to the punch with a bunch of wet snow last night—not a great deal, but enough for someone at the Villa Walther (why do I suspect the Wests with their twins?) to make a snowman and me to go out and buy some gloves for Brady and me. Mittens for Ned are less of an issue since we realized that he can fit the cast neatly into the sleeve of my warm jacket, which, as an extra perk, completely covers both of his hands. I also got myself a chic hat and a scarf. Fortunately both boys have and will wear the hats Peter gave them last year for Xmas—good for Uncle Peter!

11/6/95

Dear Rick,

. . . Big interest for me has been cutting Ned's nails. I had to do it before the surgery under orders from Big Nurz, did it again last night because he was growing such talons. As I did the deed I realized that the nails on the casted arm were twice as long as those on the free one! Gives me a sense that his body is apportioning its resources and a strong cheery feeling of his health and resilience. He can now crook his little finger against mine and give a creditable pull. YES!

11/6/95

Dear Joan . . .

On Ned's nails, does the ratio of lengths indicate how much the active hand naturally wears down its nails? . . .

11/6/95

Dear Rick,

Someone else at lunch suggested the wear-and-tear thesis, but I'm not buying it! I much prefer my vital spirits. . . .

11/8/95

Dear Rick,

I'm gearing up for another day of reading—soon it is going to be time for me to start pulling together for a focus. Boys are both fine. As far as I can tell Julie is fast becoming an item in Brady's life—at least phone conversations have suddenly become hours' long and private. I have no one else who is interested in reaching me telephonically so I'm just letting it go. Ned is as full of beans as ever—amazing to me how he has just accepted this cast as part of the landscape and gets on with things—an inspiration.

11/9/95

Dear Rick,

Trying to get to work, but first I write to you. Brady had a German lesson here yesterday and it's hard to tell whether he or the teacher enjoyed it more, so that seems a good thing. I've got to keep working to set one up for Ned, but he is young and so needs a different teacher. Last night was a bit compli- cated. I invited a *Kolleg* philosopher who left his family in England (us in reverse) for dinner. Just as he arrived we got a call from the Wests saying that both Beth and Christopher had the flu and could we please let them rest by taking the twins for a couple of hours. So we did, a great time was had by all, and the apartment looks as if it was hit by a bomb. Through it all we managed to get Ned's spelling assignment done, so perhaps we are beginning to get our feet on the ground. Brady is meanwhile so extra-ordinarily happy— whether because of Julie or his projected good report card or his triumphant German lesson or what I can't say—that it's a lift to live with him. Ned is also on the up and up. All we need is you and you are coming soon. Maybe that's why we are all so cheery. In any case I hope you can borrow some of the cheer for your day.

So day by day we moved into the city and our new lives within it. Periodically I would have to make an appointment to see Dr. Waldemeyer or ask him a question. It was a refreshingly direct process.

> *"Guten Tag. Sie haben die Nummer 555 31 18 in Berlin gewählt. Hinterlassen Sie bitte eine Nachricht. Ich rufe Sie bald möglich zurück. Vielen Dank."*
>
> ["Good day. You have dialed number 555 31 18 in Berlin. Please leave a message. I will call you back as soon as possible. Many thanks."]
>
> "Hello, this is Joan Richards, Ned's mother. Would you please call me at 555 18 81? Thank you."

"Waldemeyer."

"Hello, Dr. Waldemeyer. Ned forgot, and put his cast in the bath this evening. I'm afraid it is wet and needs to be changed. I'm sorry to bother you with such a trivial problem, but I do not know who else to call or how to handle it."

"Don't worry, Mrs. Richards. It happens all the time. Bring him to the *Gipsraum* tomorrow morning at nine. I make sure someone is there to look at it for you."

Our appointments with the surgeon, three in six weeks, were reassuring. He was pleased with his handiwork and the X rays showed that all of the parts of Ned's elbow were where they ought to be. After two weeks the stitches were removed through a hole in the cast; after four weeks Waldemeyer checked it with another X ray and was pleased with the way it looked.

As the first of December approached there were two challenges—the operation for Dr. Waldemeyer and the six-month follow-up MRI for Dr. Jennings. The first seemed well under control: "We take out the pins. Then we try to move it," Dr. Waldemeyer said. For the follow-up MRI, I contacted a pediatrician who arranged for an appointment in the week following the surgery.

Rick's Thanksgiving visit was to fall in the week before Dr. Waldemeyer wanted to remove Ned's pins. I tried not to be impatient about a scheduling issue that meant I would lose two weeks of work time just as I was building up a head of steam. It was in many ways better from the family point of view that the inconvenient three-day hospitalization the Germans required not interrupt our time together. The procedure was surgically trivial, comparable in magnitude to a tooth extraction. It was not really important that Rick be there.

11/14/95

Dear Rick,

I do have the information about your time of arrival and we will be there with bells on. Ned said last night: "I wish Dad was here." It was great to say: "He will be soon."

11/17/95

Dear Joan,

See you tomorrow! I am going to try to smuggle in fresh cranberries as well as two varieties of canned, in case they impound the fresh. I am not in great shape, probably due to not sleeping well and work pressure. I look forward to a safe haven, albeit brief.

It was wonderful to have Rick with us again. Ned's operation had granted us an unexpected stepping-stone across what had looked like a long time apart, so it was quite natural to have him around. We had a pleasant week together punctuated by a quiet sixteenth birthday party for Brady. Someone among his newfound friends gave him a card pointing out that were he in the States this would spell a driver's license, but he did not seem to mind too much. Two days later we hosted a sprawling Thanksgiving dinner populated by a motley crew of isolated Americans. It was reminiscent of graduate student feasts and we found much to be thankful for as we ate the turkey with cranberry and pumpkin pie that Rick had smuggled across the Atlantic. It was hard that he was always coming and going, but we seemed to be managing all right, and his next visit, for Christmas, was in less than six weeks.

Ein Paar Tage (A Few Days)

On Monday Rick flew off and the boys went back to school. I busily put together a commentary for a seminar Rudolf gave at the Max Planck Institute on Wednesday. On Thursday Ned had to check in to the hospital. I held in mind an image of the clear, straight bones of the X ray pictures, marred only by the startlingly large metallic pins in them. Still the open-endedness of Dr. Waldemeyer's phrase, "then we try to move it," began to haunt me.

It was impossible to separate my fears for Ned's elbow from my dread of returning to the nothingness of motherhood on Station H. I was just building my momentum at the *Wissenschaftskolleg* and really did not want to interrupt the process. I made sure that Ned would have a bed on the ward itself, in hopes that the presence of other children and their parents would help to pass the time. I took more assertive action as well. The operation was scheduled for a Friday and Dr. Waldemeyer had been vague about when Ned could come home. "How long? I don't know. *Ein paar Tage.* A few days." It wasn't specific enough to be clear that Ned wouldn't be simply warehoused over the weekend. I called Dr. Waldemeyer to get his assurance that he would release Ned on Saturday, before he and all other effective medical personnel disappeared.

The doctor was reluctant to commit himself: "Once a child goes home, it is hard to readmit him."

"But you aren't going to have to readmit him, are you? You are just taking out pins!"

"Yes, but maybe he should stay longer to move his arm."

"He doesn't have to be in a hospital to exercise his arm!"

"Mrs. Richards." The doctor was irritated. "You can always do what you want. I cannot stop you. You can always sign for him and take him home. You can be responsible."

"But, Dr. Waldemeyer. You must see that I can't do that! I have already made one major error in judgment about this case. I can't do something now against your orders. You have to help me here."

"Mrs. Richards. It is very difficult for me to tell you what to do. I check on Ned after my lecture on Saturday. We decide then."

Thursday, I made our way through the now somewhat familiar procedure of check-in. Because the anesthesiologist's trailer closed at one o'clock we had to begin at noon. We went first to the *Aufnahme* to register, then to the anesthesiologist to discuss the procedure, to the *Gipsraum* to exchange Ned's cast for a splint, to the X-ray department for a new set of pictures. Altogether the procedures took about an hour, the waiting between two and three. By four o'clock Ned was perched on one of three beds in *Zimmer Eins* of Station H.

It was a poorly designed space for visitors; the only place that a parent might sit was at the foot of the bed. Ned was in the bed by the door and another child, Nils, was in the middle bed. The bed by the window was empty. Nils's mother was sitting at the end of Nils's bed. Were I to do the same I would have blocked her ability to come and go. I brought a chair in by the sink so I could be out of her way and closer to Ned's head. The nurses frowned on this arrangement because they wanted clear access to the water, but I just moved when they were present and feigned incomprehension at their more general comments.

Nils and Ned plunged cheerfully into a German card game. As the boys bumbled their way through Nils's explanation of the rules, I could see in action the way schoolchildren learn foreign languages. It is more difficult for self-conscious adults, but Nils's mother and I chatted over the foot of Ned's bed. I told her a bit about Ned's elbow; she told me about the elusive infection in Nils's hip that had led him to be hospitalized for observation. Her tale was interesting and my linguistic challenge formidable, but even as I struggled to find the proper noun, remember its gender, fix its case, or conjugate a verb, most of me was waiting for Dr. Waldemeyer.

My attention had been fixed during a brief encounter when he had whisked through a room where Ned and I were waiting for something or another. "*Sooo!*" he had said, his hair flying, his eyes resting on Ned's arm now bound by a mere Ace bandage to the bottom of his cast. "I have no time now, but we see whether you can move it tonight! I see you later."

Half an hour passed, then another, then another. It was pitch dark outside and quite dark in the room because Nils's mother objected to overhead lighting and the individual bedlights were weak. Ned and Nils were both restless, Nils because nothing ever happened, Ned because he knew that the next day something certainly would. They circled their dinners of dreary cold cuts, and quickly rejected them in favor of candy from Nils's father, who dropped in after work. After about an hour the man left. I dared not leave the bed for even a minute for fear of missing Dr. Waldemeyer. On my digital watch, the witching hour of seven, when parents were supposed to leave the floor, clicked closer and closer. I paced the corridor.

At about six-forty-five, Dr. Waldemeyer arrived. He was tired. Eyes dull, grin forced, feet positively flat in their tennis shoes, he braced himself to face the mothers on the floor. Countless *Frauen,* frantic from hours of waiting, poured upon him from all of the rooms on Station H. Ned's was the first bed. "Well, my dear, how is your arm?" the doctor asked.

Nils's mother swooped. "*Wie gut!*" she cried. "*Ich habe den ganzen Tag gewartet und Sie sprechen Englisch!* That's a good one! I have waited all day and you speak English!" Two mothers from the adjoining room joined in her protest. The doctor capitulated and switched to German. Nils's mother launched into her concerns about Nils. A woman with long black hair scrambled to get the doctor to look at the incision in her son's knee. A mousy one wanted to know when her son could come home.

Even had I been linguistically able I had no desire to increase to four the number of women competing for one man's attention. I retreated with Ned into a game of Rummy. By the time it was over the doctor was gone. Ned was cheerfully ready to follow Nils's lead into the world of German television, leaving his left arm comfortably motionless in its splint. I kissed him good night and promised to be there when he came back from his operation the next day.

The next morning I got to the hospital promptly at eight-thirty. Ned was already gone. I had known he would be, but despite all of my rational insistences about the triviality of the procedure I was not confident enough to stay away. Nils was off somewhere, so I sat alone in *Zimmer Eins* reading Brady's text copy of *Hamlet.* It was a last-minute grab from among the rather slim pickings in the apartment, more appealing than Berlin guidebooks or German grammar texts.

In the event it was a wonderful choice. I sat in the Otto-Hoffen-Heim and drank in Shakespeare's English. It was like a nectar that nourished my sense of self against the drain of all the German with which I was surrounded and to which I was trying to conform. I marveled at its poetry and at the ways in which Shakespearean expression permeates our current speech. There were tiny things: "will he nill he" which has turned into the "willy-nilly" I can never find in dictionaries; the larger expressions "it is a custom more honored in the breach," "the time is out of joint," "the slings and arrows of outrageous fortune;" the inevitable sexism, "frailty, thy name is woman;" and those phrases longer yet that still tantalize interpreters: "There are more things on heaven and earth, Horatio/Than are dreamed of in your philosophy." I sat in the empty German hospital room and reveled in my language like a pig in mud.

At about ten-thirty Ned was wheeled back to the room. His arm looked exactly the same, wrapped to its half cast by the Ace bandage. He did not look too different either; it was a great relief to see that the anesthesiologist had really been able to administer such a light anesthetic that it left him hardly groggy at all. Soon the man himself arrived, to check on his patient. He had carefully washed and packaged the pins from Ned's arm so Ned could have them, and was as pleased as I with Ned's cheerful alertness. He and Ned bantered happily together in a German/English patois. To me, however, he made it clear that he was not an orthopedist. All he could say to my questions about movement was *"Ich weiss es nicht.* I don't know."

After he left, Ned and I played cards for a while. At about noon, Nils reappeared from the *Spielzimmer,* or gameroom, where he had spent the morning. He and Ned were glad to see each other and plunged into their card game. There was no sign of Dr. Waldemeyer, the nurses were absolutely unable to predict his actions, and I was hungry. So I stepped out for a bite to eat.

Actually, stepped out is a misnomer for the process involved in my getting lunch. It took at least two hours to catch the 110 bus, ride to the end of the appropriate *See,* walk to the *Wissenschaftskolleg,* eat lunch, and then reverse the trip. The procedure was somewhat elaborate by any measure, but the hospital cafeteria was closed to all but hospital personnel during lunchtime, and the only other identifiable eatery was a small *Imbiss* whose menu I'd exhausted in Ned's previous hospital stay. Besides, it was important for my sense of self to maintain my professional identity even if the best I could do was a hurried lunch.

On this particular day I paid a high price for my independence. When I returned, I found I had missed both the physical therapist and Dr. Waldemeyer. Ned sat cheerily in bed, his arm again securely splinted. "I could move it!" he said. It was wonderful to hear his report, but I did not dare unwrap the arm to experiment myself. All afternoon I waited for the doctor to return.

Nils's mother was also there, still worrying about Nils's frustratingly persistent infection. His being in the hospital meant that she had to leave his younger brother with a neighbor while she sat in *Zimmer Eins*. It completely disrupted her family life. Apparently the latest word was that Nils would be kept in the hospital at least one more week. His mother was making the best of it by decorating the room for St. Nicholas Day, on December 6. This afternoon she was engaged in laboriously constructing a large, stellated polyhedron from multicolored quantities of paper cones.

Room decoration, craft projects, and minor celebrations have never been my forte. I was not invited to Germany to twist carefully cut paper triangles into cones and, following strict instructions, to fashion them into a large prickly ball. I did not come 4,000 miles from home to wield blunt scissors in a semidark room of restless children that was periodically invaded by nurses who pointed out I was in the way.

Still, I was acutely aware that it did not lighten Nils's mother's load that Ned and I didn't even know that the coming Wednesday was St. Nicholas Day, or that my nontechnical German was so bad that it took several tries to get across that on this day children put out their shoes for candy or coal from the saint. I tried to atone for my failings by cutting triangles efficiently.

"*Aber nein! Das ist zuviel Rotes!* But no! That is too many red ones!"

I reminded myself that the woman was as frustrated as I. "*Es tut mir leid.* I'm sorry," I said and relinquished my scissors.

All afternoon I tried to be as unobtrusive as possible among the frustrated mothers on Station H. Dr. Waldemeyer held the keys to each of our predicaments but his appearances among us were completely random. This meant we were trapped in a world in which the smooth-flowing time measured by our watches was meaningless. Mother time on Station H moved in fits and starts; it was measured by the length of chapters, of card games, the attention spans of ten-year-olds, the patience levels of their mothers. Newton gave no credence to chaotic time like this. Both his absolute and his relative times were regular and linearly structured. For Newton, Station H time did not exist; he literally defined it out of the world.

As I alternately shuffled cards, sorted cones, stammered through conversation, and paced, I certainly empathized with Newton's desire to do away with chaotic time. Around me the other mothers snapped at one another, at their children, at me. We all wiggled under the discipline of Station H like De Morgan's Alice under the discipline of the comb.

By about six-thirty, I had reached the end of every rope I had. It was plain that Dr. Waldemeyer had made his only visit when I was at lunch, and I could not stand the darkling room another moment. Nils was turning his attention to the television and I knew Ned would happily do the same. I kissed him good night and Nils's mother kissed Nils. Then she gave me a ride home.

The next day I arose early so I could do my shopping on the way to picking up Ned. When I got to the hospital at about nine-thirty he was still cheerful. Apparently Dr. Waldemeyer had visited him as soon as I left and had again released the arm so Ned could show him how it moved. He was appreciative, Ned reported, but had told Ned he had to move his arm a lot. He could not do so at present, though, because it was once again bound to its splint. Nils's mother was presumably shopping; Nils was deep in German cartoons, which bored even Ned. I dealt a hand of rummy.

Two-and-a-half hours later, when Dr. Waldemeyer arrived, he was accompanied by a couple of other doctors in street clothes. One of them unwrapped Ned's arm and stood aside so we could watch him move it. Happily Ned flexed his scrawny little arm and it moved—a little, *very* little, only about forty degrees of arc. It was pathetic, but Ned saw only the improvement over his previous total immobility. He smiled.

Dr. Waldemeyer did not. He turned to me. "It's not very good," he said. "He must move it. It is very important. You may go now, but he must come back on Monday." He prepared to leave, followed by his minions.

I would not let him go. "I need ten minutes of your time," I said. "I can see you don't have it right now. Tell me when you do and I'll be there."

He was startled. "I must go now," he said. "I come back in half an hour."

I did not wait for him to return. Instead I went back downstairs and lurked in the hall outside his office. Students and doctors I recognized from here and there straggled out one by one. As the stream dwindled, I checked with one to see that Dr. Waldemeyer was still within. "Oh, yes!" the young man said and went to fetch him.

Soon thereafter Dr. Waldemeyer appeared and I began to work my way through a list of questions that had been building for weeks. I asked about the *Ulnar Epicondyle,* its relation to epiphyses and to growth. I asked about the nerves of the arm, their relation to movement and dexterity. I asked about ligaments, tendons, and muscles. The questions led

Dr. Waldemeyer into his element; we stood in the hall outside his office extending and flexing our arms, comparing elbow angles, and wiggling fingers. I was his only audience. He did not issue a single command. We were both happy.

Against the background of the mini-lecture we turned to the particular challenge of Ned's elbow. Elbow movement is measured as if on a protractor, where zero is total extension and 180 degrees would represent total bending toward the shoulder; most adults have between 150 and 170 degrees of flexion. With Ned under the general anesthetic, Dr. Waldemeyer had been able to move my son's arm from about 40 degrees to about 130 degrees, which, though rather restricted, the doctor considered adequate. While awake, however, Ned could move it only from about 45 degrees to about 85 degrees. More was impossibly painful, because the muscles and tendons were tight and constricted after months in a cast. Movement was very important, however, to loosen the joint and prevent the formation of inhibiting scar tissue. Ned needed intensive physical therapy, two hours a day, until he could move the arm. Otherwise it might never move more than it did at present.

In this effort, Dr. Waldemeyer was clear that the most important motion was flexion, which is motion toward the shoulder. Extension, the ability to hold one's arm straight, is an aesthetic issue, he explained, holding his arms out as if a ballet dancer. Flexion, on the other hand, is useful. He mimed buttoning a shirt, eating an apple, scratching the back of his neck and the small of his back. When he was awake, Ned's flexion was not even 90 degrees; Dr. Waldemeyer wanted at least the 130 degrees he had been able to reach under general anesthetic.

Children respond very differently to pain, the man explained, so it was hard to predict how long this would take. He seemed to be thinking in terms of several weeks, which chilled my blood. He was honoring our agreement by letting Ned go home for the weekend, but it was imperative that on Monday Ned be back on Station H to start his regime. Reluctantly I agreed, but there was the problem of his scheduled MRI. When I explained the issue Dr. Waldemeyer was instantly helpful: "I write a recipe for Dr. Geisler. He does it here."

Station H

Journal, I'm thankful for:
I'm thankful for a good house and a little money. It's because a lot of people can't even eat a good meal. I can go to Germany for a year and still live under a roof. I'm glad to have a good education and am able to go to school. I'm also thankful for the people who care enough to come to my birthday party and give me something. I'm also thankful that I'm in good medical condition and not on the verge of death because I want to live outside of a hospital a lot of my life.

Ned Richards

I found Ned's school-assigned Thanksgiving piece on Friday evening as I was cleaning for his hospital homecoming. It made me all the more secure about the decision that led us out of the Otto-Hoffen-Heim and onto the 110 bus that chilly afternoon. It was the day before the first Sunday in Advent and outdoor *Weihnachtsmärkte*, Christmas bazaars, were springing up around the city. Ned spied one, and his eyes lit up like the Christmas lights.

"Oh, let's get one of those wreaths with candles!"

We scooted back and down the stairs of the bus to buy the last Advent wreath from a couple shivering at the back of their truck. "It's made of real branches and look! there are little pinecones!" Ned enthused as the woman wrapped it for him. I added his bag of clothes to my burden of groceries so he could carry his treasure. It balanced on the shelf of his two arms; he held it with his mittened right hand, leaving the casted left one buried for warmth in his jacket sleeve.

Cheery and triumphant we made our way toward the Villa Walther. Our impulse buy had added at least a half mile to the trek, but Ned chattered happily as we walked along. We discussed St. Nicholas Day, which Nils had told him about; he was gleeful as he contemplated the windfall of an extra chance for goodies just because he was in Germany.

By the time we turned into the path beside the *See* we had been walking for about half an hour. With Racky peeking from his knapsack, the Advent wreath balanced on his arms, Ned was getting tired. So was I as I juggled several bags of groceries in each arm. We proceeded single file into the woods; Ned moving ahead down the familiar path while I trundled along behind. Suddenly he slid on a patch of ice. He twisted frantically as he went down to land on his right side. His casted left arm was safe; his right, with the wreath lay beneath him. Terrified, I raced to him as he sobbed on the frozen ground.

"The wreath is broken! It's ruined! The candles are broken!" he cried. It was true that a protruding candle was broken at its base.

"Don't worry, Neddy." I helped him to his feet. "It will be just fine. We can get new candles."

"But it was so pretty! It was perfect!" he wailed.

"We'll make it pretty again," I promised.

It was not enough. The little boy who had been so perky minutes before was now weak, injured, and deeply sad. He clung to me as I brushed him off. I tucked the wreath under my arm, put all of my bags in my right hand, and held Ned's mitten with my left as we resumed our walk. Silently we walked the rest of the way to the Villa Walther.

It was a subdued afternoon. I had had no qualms as we marched out of the Otto-Hoffen-Heim; I was completely secure in the knowledge that in America we would have been sent home the same day as the operation. But Ned's fall had frightened me; I realized how little I knew about his postoperative condition. I could see I had overestimated his strength. What else did I not know about? When he let me take my son home Dr. Waldemeyer had merely been acceding to the demands of a determined mother. Did he think I knew what I was doing? Were there instructions I would have been given in America? I certainly couldn't call him to ask. I kept a watchful eye on Ned who lay reading on the amorphous couch.

Sunday was a good day. Ned and I spent much of it with Clare in a *Weihnachtsmarkt* just around the corner. We bought new candles for the Advent wreath, Ned dipped one of his own and we ate *Rostbratwurst* and *Nudeln* while listening to a brass band, a bit out of tune because of the cold. But behind the façade of my Christmas cheer, I was being torn apart by the contradiction between my commitment to Ned and my commitment to work. I had come to Germany determined to make up for lost time, but despite my best efforts to control it, Ned's elbow had been a major focus of attention ever since I'd arrived.

Dr. Waldemeyer called that evening to make sure we were clear about Ned's situation. As we talked, I tried to take matters in hand. He and I were at essentially the same professional level, as measured by the German university system, and though in very different fields with different sets of criteria for advancement, it required no great leap for either of us to understand the other on this level. The doctor was absolutely clear that Ned needed to return to the hospital but had emphasized that Ned would be fine alone—they would teach him his lessons, he would have physical therapy, they had a playroom. I decided to leave him to them.

I went a step further and took on the question of time directly. I explained to Dr. Waldemeyer that I found it difficult to wait for him in the hospital, and provided a long and comprehensive list of numbers he could use to reach me. If I wanted to reach him, I would leave a message on his machine. This way I could control my time. I could work until about four, walk to the 4:23 bus, and spend the time from five to seven with Ned as opposed to waiting for his doctor. It seemed a good plan.

Monday morning, Ned and I boarded the 110 bus in order to reach *Zimmer Eins* by eight-thirty. Nils was still there, glad to see Ned back. Ned was cheery; it seemed that he might rather enjoy his day on Station H. He looked up from his card game with Nils to grin as I crisply left.

It was good to get out of the Otto-Hoffen-Heim, though it would be wrong to say that I got into my work. I got into my office but my Victorians seemed very far away. Besides Ned was sick enough for my taste; I couldn't face Ellis.

I did, however, have another little project that had grown out of my hospital Shakespeare reading. In the last lines of Act 2, Hamlet is wondering whether he can trust his father's ghost.

> . . . The spirit that I have seen
> May be a devil, and the devil hath power
> T'assume a pleasing shape, yea, and perhaps
> Out of my weakness and my melancholy,
> As he is very potent with such spirits,
> Abuses me to damn me. I'll have grounds
> More relative than this. The play's the thing
> Wherein I'll catch the conscience of the king.

I've often heard the line "Abuses to damn me" and the one about "the play's the thing" is almost a platitude. But it was the forgotten sentence between them that caught my eye in the Otto-Hoffen-Heim. "I'll have grounds/ More relative than this."

What struck me was the word *relative*. I'd always thought it was a weak word. Newton's relative time and relative space were the just the best mere humans could do in the face of absolutes; they were reflections of human weakness and limitation. But in this passage Hamlet looks toward the relative as a position of strength, and he explicitly juxtaposes its power against the possibility that he might be misled by his personal limitations and prejudices. It carried none of the wishy-washy overtones I routinely attached to the word. In the hospital I had checked the glossary of Brady's edition: "relative: closely related to fact." It was a start, but it left me still unsure about the range of implications of the word.

Now in my office I could investigate further. I looked up the Leibniz-Clarke correspondence. Their world was closer to Shakespeare's than to mine, but I thought that Leibniz had there used *relative* as weakly as Newton and I did: "I hold space to be something merely relative." But that morning, I noticed something I'd never seen before. The correspondence between the German and the Englishman had originally been in French, which was the international intellectual language of the time. I was reading an English translation that Clarke published a year after Leibniz's death, which is universally recognized as the definitive translation. I'd never paid particular attention to its technicalities, but this morning I noticed a footnote to the word *merely*. At the bottom of the page the modern editor indicated that in Leibniz's original French the word was *purement*, purely. "I hold space to be something purely relative."

I was amazed. "Purely relative" was a powerful phrase; by translating it as "merely relative" his English antagonist had trivialized it. Leibniz's space was not *merely* relative; it was not a pale imitation of an unattainable absolute. Leibniz's space was *purely* relative, wholly and unabashedly relative.

I thought again about what this meant. On the one hand, not very much. Leibniz's rejection of Newton's absolutes did not mean that he disagreed with Newton about basic facts; inertial balls rolled through his world just as they did through Newton's. The difference lay at a deeper level, at the level of the basic principles on which these laws rested. Although Leibniz agreed with Newton in the way he described motion, he argued to his conclusions from a different set of assumptions.

This difference is not trivial, because their view of motion required some argument; it is not immediately evident from our experience that a moving object will move forever unless something impedes it. Rolling balls do not roll on forever, and hockey pucks slide to a halt. To establish that these stoppings are not essential, that they are due to essentially trivial though unavoidable circumstances, required considerable argument.

Absolute space would support Newton's argument, which might go like this: Because it is infinite and essentially undifferentiated, in absolute space there is no way to tell the difference between an object moving along in a straight line and an object at rest. There are no trees to mark one's passage, there is no wind to blow one's hair, and so in absolute space, motion and rest are essentially indistinguishable from each other. That this is the truth in absolute space signaled to Newton that it was the underlying truth in our relative space as well. In our common experience, being in motion and being at rest may seem very different, but in physics we must always be careful not to make essential distinctions between them, because in absolute space these distinctions do not exist.

Obliterating the distinction between motion and rest leads virtually immediately to the inertial law. We all know that a ball at rest remains at rest unless something moves it; if motion is just like rest, this leads directly to the conclusion that a ball in motion must remain in motion unless something stops it. In Newton's world, this kind of argument from absolute space was enough to establish the truth of the inertial law in the teeth of all of our experience with objects that stop. In Newton's view, behind the mere appearances of our world lies an absolute reality, a mathematical reality in which the inertial law holds.

Leibniz did not disagree about the truth of the inertial law, but he did disagree about absolute space. He did not believe that it existed, and he could find the inertial law without it. He could draw his conclusions from considering the purely relative world of experience. The key was to approach that world from different perspectives. In the case of the inertial law, he might consider the perspective of a person drifting down a river on a barge, and that of someone standing on the shore. The person on the barge is used to considering the trees and houses that she or he passes as fixed; this is what makes it clear the barge is moving. However, assuming that it is a calm day and the barge is moving uniformly, there is nothing else in the barge-person's experience to indicate that he or she is moving; she or he could pour drinks, play catch, or ever play billiards on the barge just as on the shore. And, on the barge as on the shore, all moving objects would eventually come to rest.

As long as they focused on their own experience, the barge-person and the shore-person might see motion and rest as essentially different. However, as soon as they tried to construct a world that encompassed both of their experiences, the distinction would break down. Balls that appear stationary to the barge-person would be moving past the person on the shore. Balls the shore-person sees as still would to the person on the barge be moving backwards. Any conversation between the two would soon make it clear that in the larger universe that included them both, there is no essential difference between motion and rest. The single world that could encompass both of their experiences would look very much like Newton's absolute space.

So, when it comes to things like the inertial law, Newton's and Leibniz's approaches yielded the same results, but there was this difference. Leibniz saw the truths of physics as deeply embedded in a variety of observations of the everyday world. When, as in the case of inertia, a fundamental law seemed to contradict everyday experience, it was not because of an unmoving absolute; it was because the law of inertia was required to make sure that all perspectives were equally valid.

To me, on leave from the world of mothers in the Otto-Hoffen-Heim, the implied value shift loomed large. I penciled in the correction and reread the passage. "As for my own opinion, I hold space to be something purely relative, as time is. For space denotes in terms of possibility, an order to things which exist at the same time, considered as existing together. . . . And when many things are seen together one perceives that order of things among themselves."

It was very satisfying to see the real resting equally on the facts of the case and the relations of the people responding to these facts. With this approach the reality for mothers in the Otto-Hoffen-Heim could be truly different from that of the doctors, or the scholars at the *Wissenschaftskolleg*. One was not intrinsically better, more accurate, or more real than the other. What was real had somehow to account for all those differences.

I held myself the whole day in my office. Tomorrow will be easier, I told myself firmly as I reviewed notes and made lists of things to do. I did not leave until four o'clock.

I got to the hospital at about four-forty-five, and as I walked past the Anesthesiology trailer, I ran into Nils's mother, who was escaping for a brief walk. "*Ach, wie gut!* Oh, good" she said. "You are here! Ned has been somewhat *unruhig*." [*Unruhig*: unhappy, discontent.] I quickened my pace.

In *Zimmer Eins* I found Ned lying determinedly on his stomach, his head buried in the pillow. When he realized that it was me, he erupted into furious tears. "Where have you been?" he howled. "I want to go home. Take me home. Take me home, now!"

I could not take Ned home. Instead I read against his fury. I had brought with me James Thurbers's *The Thirteen Clocks,* and he led us into his fairytale world of good and evil negotiated by the Golux, a little person who "wore an indescribable hat, whose eyes were wide and astonished, as if everything were happening for the first time."

"'Who are you?' the minstrel asked.

"'I am the Golux,' said the Golux, proudly, 'the only Golux in the world, and not a mere Device. . . . I make mistakes, but I am on the side of Good, by accident and happenchance.'"

Ned looked at me. "Just like you," I said. "You are on the side of good but you seem to have had quite an accident!"

I read on about his mother, "a witch, but rather mediocre in her way. When she tried to turn a thing to gold, it turned to clay; and when she changed her rivals into fish, all she ever got was mermaids."

Ned laughed out loud.

After a bit more reading, Ned could talk about his problems on Station H. Physical therapy accounted for only a couple of hours, the tutoring was only half an hour, the *Spielzimmer* was filled with games that lacked crucial pieces, Big Nurz was insufferable, and Nils was slim pickings for a lifetime's companionship. There was now another boy, Peter, in the room, who seemed more Ned's type. However, Nils's bed separated them. Besides, Peter would never play because his mother read to him in German for hours on end. In fact, everyone else had a mother who put in hours by her child's bedside—the day was simply unbearable without this support.

Dr. Waldemeyer called as soon as I got home; as he put it, "Station H is a hard place for an American child." We agreed to try leaving Ned on the ward during the day and letting him spend nights at home. I was startled at the boldness of the plan, but Dr. Waldemeyer was impatient with my timidity. He acknowledged that the nurses would not like it, but they would do as he said. Perhaps this was the answer.

The next morning I made the trek to and from the hospital to take Ned to his MRI and tell him of our plan. The MRI was relatively painless with Dr. Geisler at the helm. It was nice to go through the process with someone Ned had met before and liked. *"It won't come back. It won't come back."* I had to modify my mantra a bit to fit it to the rhythm of the machine. After about forty-five minutes Ned returned to Station

H. Knowing that he would be going home at the end of the day made the whole situation infinitely more bearable, though, so I caught the 110 bus back to the *Wissenschaftskolleg*. The seminar was on Greek philology.

At four o'clock I set out to collect Ned from the Otto-Hoffen-Heim. I was lucky to find the same long-haired doctor who had talked to me the very first day we had come looking for Dr. Waldemeyer; she was one of the many anonymous doctors who swarmed occasionally, and she just happened to be on Station H when I wanted to take Ned. When I asked her how it was done, she was stunned and called Dr. Waldemeyer.

Dr. Waldemeyer's power was awesome. After he had spoken, leaving Station H was absurdly easy. We simply put on Ned's street clothes, his coat, and his indescribable hat. Then we left all of his books, games, and pajamas neatly in his little locker and walked out to catch the bus. Ned was cheery about his day and willing to continue in this commuting regime. I was triumphant.

The next morning it became clear that I had triumphed too soon. I brought Ned in at eight o'clock as agreed, so he could slip unobtrusively into the hospital schedule. It was before even parental visiting hours, so I faded out of the picture as soon as he had changed into pajamas and gotten on the bed. I did not leave the hospital, though, because I wanted to help him organize homework projects; we had agreed on this strategy as a defense against the hated *Spielzimmer*. I stood on the landing and looked at the frozen ground where I had seen the fox, almost two months before. I hoped she was warm in a den somewhere nearby, with her tail on her nose.

My reverie did not last for long. A stream of doctors, including Dr. Waldemeyer, began flowing up the stairs. It seemed that Wednesday mornings, or at least this Wednesday morning, was grand rounds. As soon as eight-thirty and visiting hours arrived, I went back to Ned. The doctors showed up about fifteen minutes later, but their coming was rather anticlimactic. They watched and mumbled when Ned demonstrated his very restricted arm motion; then they left.

In the hall I was waylaid by Big Nurz, who was surprisingly mellow, all things considered. She explained that the commuting system simply would not work, not because of her intransigence, but because of the other mothers. Apparently, Ned's leaving the night before had fomented a parental rebellion on Station H. Nils's mother, Peter's mother, and the mothers from the other rooms as well had wanted to know why their children could not go home too. Their being German did not prevent them from feeling the pressures Ned had so clearly expressed. Big Nurz clapped the fingers to the thumb of her right hand to emphasize the force of their complainings.

Although I was supportive of the other mothers standing up for themselves and their children, I could see that they were not my current concern, which was Ned. To my great relief, Big Nurz rejected the idea of bringing him back on the floor as a regular patient; she was turning her attention to getting him the requisite physical therapy on an outpatient basis. He would spend this day on Station H, but at the end of it he would go home for good. I was elated, as was Ned when I told him the news. As I left he was sitting cross-legged on the bed doing a vocabulary assignment. In the hall, Dr. Waldemeyer was standing on one foot and rotating the other, explaining to Big Nurz the musculature involved in Peter's operation.

I did not return to Station H that day. Instead, in a fierce symbolic burst of independence, I entrusted Ned's homecoming to a variety of friends and baby-sitters and went to the Max Planck Institute to hear Liza's seminar. I had been looking forward to it for months. I found it hard to keep my mind on her presentation though. My little boy was sick. How could I just leave him on his own?

When I got home, I found that my uneasiness was not wholly unfounded; all had not remained tranquil in my absence. Soon after I left, Ned had galvanized Station H by refusing medication. The precipitating issue was the persistent stiffness in Ned's arm. Apparently it was clear to the doctors on rounds that it hardly moved at all and that improvement since the operation was negligible. In response they decided to give him a painkiller before physical therapy sessions in hopes that if the arm hurt less, he could move it more.

They had not explained this to me or Ned, however. Ned was as well educated as I could make him about the implications of his being on Tegretol and the importance of his being careful about mixing medications. So, when Big Nurz arrived with the painkiller, he refused to take it. I wish I could have been a fly on the wall for this confrontation. Big Nurz was formidable, but Ned can be equally so. He avenged us all, and his own captive self, when he refused to take the medicine she offered.

She left the room and called for reinforcements, which soon congregated around Ned's bed. Many nurses, the physical therapists, and anonymous doctors gathered, in Ned's words, "to practice their English." They explained that there would be no trouble mixing this medication with the one that he already took. They emphasized its critical importance to his progress in physical therapy. Most powerful of all, they invoked the authority of Dr. Waldemeyer. The mighty name shook Ned's resolve, but he could not simply back down. "I can't decide when all of you are standing there," he said. The mass of medical authority left. About fifteen minutes later a very junior nurse arrived alone with Ned's medication. Ned took it.

I must confess that I grinned when Ned told me this tale. His spirit had not been squelched by his experiences on Station H.

"Here is the medicine, Mom. They said I'm supposed to take fifteen drops half an hour before physical therapy." Ned gave me a bottle and its accompanying literature.

"Was it OK when you took it today? How did it make you feel?"

"It gave me a headache."

"Where?" I asked, fearful that he would indicate the area of his tumor headaches. But he pointed to his temple and I could put that issue down.

"I'll check it out after dinner," I promised.

After supper, I pored over the medical circular, German dictionary at the ready. It seemed like a very strong painkiller but I could not figure out much beyond that. Even in English I am not a pharmacist. The telephone rang.

"Oh! Dr. Waldemeyer. Thank you for calling!"

"Ned had some trouble on Station H, today. He did not want to take the medicine I prescribed."

"Yes. I'm sorry that he caused trouble. He was upset about taking something new. He was worried because of his Tegretol."

"Yes, he was!" The doctor chuckled. Ned's performance had been memorable. "But you can tell him there is no trouble to mix the drops with Tegretol. They are completely different."

I asked about the headache. "No," Dr. Waldemeyer responded, "they do not give him headache. I hope they make less pain so he moves his arm."

"That would be good."

"Yes, I think it works! Yesterday he was only 90 degrees in physical therapy. Today he has 95 degrees with the drops. I hope he has 5 degrees more every day. Then I see you in a week. I want him to have 130 degrees next Wednesday."

"Oh! That would be great!"

"He should have it," the doctor said hopefully.

"Good. Thank you for calling. I'm sorry for the trouble."

"I think it is good that Ned takes responsibility."

"I do too, but it can be a bother."

"Well, no one has ever refused *Schwester* Elisabeth before."

We were both laughing as we hung up.

"Was he mad at me?" Ned asked.

"No. He understood why you were worried about the Tegretol. He says there should not be any problem with the drops, though."

"OK." Ned smiled.

"Oh, and Ned! I found out Big Nurz's name! It's Elisabeth, *Schwester* Elisabeth because she's a nurse."

"Oh, I knew that," he said. "That's what Nils calls her. But I think Big Nurz is better."

Ned settled peacefully down to his homework while I washed the dishes. Having choices is not the same as being free, I decided; when you are in a tight place what you need is support.

07.xii.1995

Dear Dr. Waldemeyer,

I want to thank you for two things, which may seem small but are important to Ned and to me. The first is for getting Ned out of the hospital as soon as possible. I realize that it was not easy. The second is for taking the trouble last night to explain the need for Ned's medication to me and through me to him. It is reassuring to find a doctor who recognizes the legitimacy of Ned's anxieties about treatment.

Gratefully yours,

Joan L. Richards

Termin (Appointment)

The next day Ned and I entered the small oasis of outpatient life among the physical therapists at the Otto-Hoffen-Heim. It took a couple of days to figure out the system, but by Monday we had it down very nicely. I would draw Ned's bath at five-forty-five so we would be ready to leave the house by six-twenty. I would waken Brady just before we left, confirm his after-school plans, and make sure he had the wherewithal to get through his day. Then Ned and I would walk out into December's morning darkness to catch the 110 bus at six-forty-three. Accurate to the minute, we would claim the coveted front seat and lumber peacefully through the sleepy streets of Berlin.

By seven o'clock we were at the Otto-Hoffen-Heim. Ned took his drops; he never again complained that they caused a headache. Then we were ready to be the first customers at the cafeteria.

At seven-thirty we went to physical therapy. It was a very different world from Station H.

"*Hallo,* Ned. I am Sigrid Sonne. You can call me Sigrid. I work with you for physical therapy."

It soon became evident that Sigrid's personal introduction signaled more than an accidental difference between physical therapists and nurses; it reflected the intense and personal experience that physical therapy entails. A typical session proceeded in two parts. In the first, Ned lay on a table while Sigrid bent and then straightened his arm as much as possible.

"Oww! That hurts!"

"Yes, it does hurt. But that is what we have to do. Try to relax. It will get better."

It was Sigrid's job to move Ned's arm until it would move no more; she was firm and determined, pushing in each direction until he yelped. Keeping the process going required that they maintain a constant constructive interaction.

"That's good, Ned! Now a little bit more."

"No, Sigrid, no more!"

"Yes, you can do it. . . . Good! We'll just hold it here a minute. It will stop hurting if we just hold it. . . . OK. Now a little bit more."

"That's enough Sigrid, that's enough!"

"OK, Ned. That's enough. I won't do any more. Just hold it." She measured the angle with her *Winkelmesser*, or orthopedic protractor [technically, a goniometer].

Table work was hard, but the second part of the session was more fun. Then Ned was allowed to use the gym and play with balls, sticks, and rubber bands; Ned's favorite was left-handed basketball. It was fun, but also frustrating; Ned struggled with the realization of how poorly he played, how often he failed to dribble the ball off the floor, how easily Sigrid intercepted it, how often his throws—by direction always two-handed—veered off to the left because the two arms were completely out of balance. But Sigrid enjoyed Ned, and so did her colleagues who often filled in when she was on vacation, ill, or otherwise not around. She had been assigned to him because she spoke English; the others simply taught him German.

By eight o'clock and the end of the session it was beginning to be light. Ned and I could see each other on opposite sides of the street as we waited to take buses in opposite directions on the Clayallee. He would raise his fist in triumph and salute when his bus came before mine.

Whoever won the first bus contest, Ned arrived at school late, but not so late he could not keep up with his classes. Mrs. Harkin was wholly supportive and he was thrilled to be back with his friends. In the afternoon, he had another physical therapy session which he handled himself. It was rather fun for him—a somewhat unusual form of after-school recreation. The whole system was quite satisfactory.

This physical therapy schedule allowed me several hours in my office every day. I was reading a correspondence between De Morgan and an Irish mathematician, William Rowan Hamilton, which had the advantage of being organized in a single volume by a nineteenth-century editor. It was convenient because easy to pick up and put down. Mostly though I put it down. I was trying to emulate De Morgan's professionalism, but the constant back and forth between the Otto-Hoffen-Heim and the *Wissenschaftskolleg*, between myself as a mother and myself as a scholar, was getting to me. I spoke to the rector about my practical problems: "Don't worry," he said. "Many fellows get off to a slow start. In a month it will be all settled and you can get back to work again."

In the meantime I struggled to keep up appearances. I listened to lecture after lecture, forcing myself to focus long enough to formulate a relevant question before the surge of language overwhelmed me; then I sat still and attentive like a well-behaved child in church. Day after day I tried to be on my best behavior at lunch, which usually meant being quiet as my colleagues spoke of their work, the latest academic controversy, Berlin politics, the latest performance at the opera or symphony.

It was not that I could not follow such things, and virtually everyone would graciously switch to English if I sat with them. My problem was that I was deeply engaged in what was happening to Ned, and there was no place for this topic anywhere. Many of the fellows had left their families at home, in far-off cities or even countries. By fiat, certainly, even the most familially devoted was not to bring the families to lunch. So most of my ruminations were inappropriate and out of place, and I knew it. I did my best to keep them to myself or send them to Rick.

12/7/95

Dear Rick,

Ned is at home and very cheery, though his arm moves very little. (Brady's response was "What a gyp!") My time seems totally eaten up by physical therapy, the 110 bus, and waiting. I am not happy about this at all, but I want Ned to be able to move the damn arm. So . . . there you have it. The beat goes on. I try not to get discouraged, but it seems a bit much.

12/8/95

Dear Rick,

Well, Ned's second day as an outpatient, and I'm concerned about how well physical therapy is working (it's not). So I think would be Dr. W., though we haven't spoken. I suspect I'll not hear anything further from him for a while. In the meantime I am going to call Dr. Lyman and ask him to call Dr. W. again. The last time this process took a couple of days. I want to get it rolling; by the time they hook up things may be clearer.

12/10/95

Dear Rick,

On the PT front, progress in the extension direction seems to be real ("*gut*"). In the crucial bending direction yesterday's physical therapist was quite clear that it is not ("*schlecht, ganz schlecht* [bad, totally bad]"). This confirms my impression. We will continue this regime until our Dr. W. appointment, Wednesday at one, but he's not going to be pleased. He has talked about putting Ned under general anesthetic again to loosen up the arm that way. I'm afraid we're in for it. Dr. W. is a man of action and he's not going to take "*ganz schlecht*" as an answer for long.

In the meantime I've toyed with asking you to drop everything and come, but talked last night to Beth West, who is a doctor and a family woman. She felt 1) Ned's arm may never be 100%, but it will not stay as bad as it now is and 2) last year's crisis was of a different order of magnitude than my current frustration about taking care of Ned and getting work done. We agreed that issues of last year's kind need you; this year's need creative solutions but they do not require anything drastic. She made sense to me, so I'm moving ahead.

Night after sleepless night I filled the hours by studying German.

Ned was also troubled. One tired night he burst into tears. "Mom, I'm sorry!" he cried. "I am really trying to move it. I am really trying to make it better!" He sat on my lap in the cowflop chair. I could feel his lashes and his tears on my neck.

"It's not your fault, Neddy. You did not know you would hurt yourself on the *Wippe*! You did not know what would happen. No one did! If they had they would not have let you jump on it."

"But it's *my* elbow," he wailed. "It's *my* elbow that doesn't work and is causing so much trouble."

"Let's look at it a different way," I tried. "In English you would talk about 'my' elbow, you would say 'My elbow hurts.' In German, though, you would talk about 'the' elbow. You would say '*Der Ellbogen tut mir weh*,' the elbow hurts me. Let's be German about this. Let's forget about *your* elbow and think about *the* elbow. *The* elbow hurts you, it hurts me, it hurts Dr. Waldemeyer, it hurts Big Nurz . . . all in different ways. We are all in this together. What makes you special is just that the elbow hurts you more."

Ned sat and thought, the toes at the end of his lengthening legs pushing inexorably through his footed pajamas. Finally he said "*Ja, der Elbogen tut mir weh.*"

"*Der Elbogen tut* UNS *weh.*" Brady spoke up from his seat at the dining room table, both showing off his German and supporting my point. "It's not just you, Ned, it is all of us who have to worry about this elbow."

"I know." Ned was not sure whether Brady was being bossy or kind.

"Don't worry, kid. It will get better."

Ned began to relax and nestled down comfortably in my arms. "It's OK, old thing. Now its time to go to bed. You'll feel better in the morning."

"That's what you always say, Mom!"

"Well, I think it's true!"

He grinned and got off my lap.

"Good night, Ned," Brady said. I tucked Ned into his bed; soon thereafter Brady retired to his. Within the hour they were both asleep.

At our Wednesday appointment Ned and I found Dr. Waldemeyer in teaching mode. His office was full of students who burrowed enthusiasticaly through Ned's files while the surgeon attempted a bilingual examination of the arm.

"*Ist die Hand verletzt?* Is the hand injured?" a student asked as Dr. Waldemeyer was telling Ned to move his fingers. "*Ja,* good," the surgeon said as they wiggled.

A woman, apparently Dr. Waldemeyer's medical peer, materialized in the doorway, and began to watch the proceedings. A student pulled out the MRI picture Dr. Geisler had taken for Dr. Jennings.

"*Nein!*" Dr. Waldemeyer barked. He seemed to find the image as upsetting as I did. "*Das ist nicht unseres. Tun Sie es zurück!* That is not ours. Put it back."

The student quickly put the picture back in its envelope and Dr. Waldemeyer took the whole to his secretary. I followed with Dr. Jennings's address.

"I read Dr. Geisler's report," the German surgeon said to me. "He found no problem."

I took a deep breath of relief, and Dr. Waldemeyer paused with me for a moment. Then we moved back into the chaos of the examining room.

"*Ist das eine Knocheninfektion?* Is this a bone infection?" one of the students asked holding up a two-month-old X ray.

"*Gibt es hier vielleicht ein Stück Knochen?* Is this perhaps a piece of bone?" another queried, looking at his picture.

Dr. Waldemeyer's responses, if there were any, were mixed with his English conversation with Ned, and mumbled ruminations on his chart. I gave up trying to figure out what was happening with the elbow and began to focus on fixing a time for a telephonic communication and getting Ned's stitches out.

Dr. Waldemeyer smiled at the hovering woman and got up. "Call me!" he said. Assuming from the linguistic clue that he meant me, I asked "When?"

"Sunday," he replied. "I go for vacation this weekend." He began to leave.

"Wait!" I cried. "Can you take the stitches out?"

He was startled. "Oh, of course! He does that," he said indicating a student, who smiled happily at having been given something to do.

"Have a good vacation," I said.

"It's only three days," Dr. Waldemeyer answered, somewhat defensively.

"Even so, you can enjoy them."

The waiting woman laughed and grinned at me.

Anruf (Telephone Call)

Four more days of physical therapy produced no improvement. "That is not good," Dr. Waldemeyer said. "Come to my office tomorrow, after physical therapy. We make new X rays."

Technically the surgeon was still on vacation, so we found him dressed in mufti; he sported a suede coat, and Ned was entranced by his leather boots. He put the new X rays on his lighted table, Ned as ever by his side. He pointed out some fuzz in the picture; a blob on each side of Ned's elbow. "Here is the problem," he said simply. "Calcification. This bit means he cannot straighten his arm. This one stops the bending."

"What do we do?" I asked.

"Operate," he said. "I do it on Thursday. I can get this on the outside through the scar. I can try to get this on the inside with *Arthoskopie*. But then," he added, "he must move it. And move it and move it." He continued pumping his arm for emphasis. "We will have to put in a *Katheter* for the *Narcoses* to kill the pain. Because Ned will have a lot of pain. You must talk to the *Anästhesist* to see if he will do it. He must move it. Otherwise he has *Ankylosis;* it gets stiff again."

Operate? I was appalled. Screwing up all my courage, I asked: "Are you sure this is what we should do? Shouldn't we get another opinion?"

"Of course," Dr. Waldemeyer said. "You have always another opinion. I must show everything to the *Chefarzt*. I do not do anything unless 'Chief' agrees." This was the first reference Dr. Waldemeyer had ever made to the Professor Mahler whose name was the only name on his stationery. Having gone through three months and two operations without any contact with said professor, he seemed to me at best a proforma personage. But Dr. Waldemeyer did not pause to further elaborate on the checks and balances of his institutional position. "We schedule this." He began the now familiar phone calls to the *Aufnahme* and to Station H. I stood silently by, my questions rendered superfluous by his crisp decisiveness.

Ned asked, somewhat fearfully, "I can go to my Christmas party tomorrow, can't I?"

"Yes." I said firmly. He relaxed.

"Don't worry, Mom," he went on, responding to my discouragement. "I know how to do this."

"Of course you do," I replied. I made an effort to pull myself together, and to smile.

When the doctor got off the phone I asked how long Ned would be in the hospital. "Oh, ten days" he responded formulaically. "I really can not let him go home with the *Katheter*. We see how long until he can move the arm."

"But are you going to be here in the week between Christmas and New Year?"

"No," he said, somewhat testily. "I have vacation. But the hospital is open. Dr. Lützen is here. He takes care of Ned."

"I see," I said, hoping I sounded cooperative. I groaned inwardly as Christmas on Station H loomed before me.

"We'll just have Christmas late!" Ned volunteered.

"You have to speak to the *Anästhesist*, though," Dr. Waldemeyer went on. "He does not usually do this on such young children. It all depends on whether he does it. Come back after ten o'clock. You can talk to him."

I remembered the anesthesiologist as a jolly young man who enjoyed practicing his rather shaky English with Ned. I doubted that our linguistic skills were up to this situation, however. At my request, Dr. Waldemeyer wrote an explanatory note to him in the little yellow notebook. "Call me tonight and tell me what he says," he said as we parted.

Numb as if under anesthesia myself, I delivered Ned to his classroom and returned to the hospital to meet with the anesthesiologist. As I had feared, the language problem loomed large. We perched on stools in Dr. Waldemeyer's examining room, writing on the examining table. He drew illustrative pictures in my notebook while explaining the issues in German.

Squinting at the figure the doctor had drawn I began to describe it back in English. "Here is the artery and here the vein. These are the nerves," I began. My nose began to bleed. I held my hand over it and made for the door. He followed and located a paper-towel dispenser. I held a towel to my nose and we continued the conversation. Blood continued to flow, soaking the towel.

"I need another towel," I admitted.

The anesthesiologist looked up from his diagram and was startled.

"Lie down," he said indicating the table.

"I'll be fine," I said, ignoring the request. "This happens when I am under pressure. I just need another towel."

He looked at me surprised. "I said, 'lie down!'" he repeated.

I realized that he meant it and that he was a doctor. I lay down. He brought me some wet towels for my nose.

He disappeared again and reappeared with a wad of wet towels in each hand. "*Heiss oder kalt?* Hot or cold?" he asked.

I was confused. "*Für das Blut,* For the blood," he explained. "On your coat."

"*Ach!*" I said. "*Kalt.*"

"*Sie sind eine Mutter.* You are a mother," he twinkled as he wiped the blood off my coat with the cold, watered towels. He chatted for a bit about his family, his five siblings and the current brood of nieces and nephews. I lay there, my toes and my nose pointing at the ceiling. His beeper went off and he went to call in the next room. "*Ich spreche mit der Mutter von einem Kind.* I am speaking to the mother of a child," I heard him say.

When he returned the young doctor allowed me to sit on the table, leaning against the wall. Our conversation returned to Ned and the situation at hand.

"Ned is a good child," he concluded after some time. "He does fine. We can do it with him."

"Thank you," I said.

He helped me off the table. My nose had stopped bleeding. We shook hands and he went to his next appointment.

My afternoon unfolded into a long series of conversations in which I broke the news to one stunned person after another. I was too overwhelmed to venture out, but the telephone enabled me to reach all over Berlin. The *Wissenschaftskolleg* agreed to provide Brady dinners for a while, Rick put into motion an emergency plan to extend his Christmas stay, friend after friend offered to come and support Ned through the long and difficult days on Station H. The situation began to assume a manageable form.

Ned came home from school full of urgency about getting a *Weihnachts* gift for the classmate whose name he had drawn from a hat. We went uptown and bought her a hand puppet as well as some decorations for the tree. When we came back I called Dr. Waldemeyer and reported the anesthesiologist's willingness to work on the project. We made an appointment for Wednesday to complete the necessary admission forms.

The next morning, Tuesday, I took Ned for a preoperative blood test, and then came back to face the *Wissenschaftskolleg* in the flesh.

Frau Breunig greeted me with a long description of ways to cheer up hospitals over Christmas. Buoyed by her suggestions I went, almost cheerful, to my office.

I turned on my computer so I could compose an e-mail message for the group of "Ned watchers" in the States who had been following Ned's progress for weeks. The phone rang.

"Dr. Waldemeyer." Over the phone the deep, gruff, Germanic voice was softened neither by frizzing hair nor gleeful smiles. "I presented Ned's case to the orthopedic group this morning, and Chief said not to operate. He said it is possible that the bones are too weak from the earlier operations. Also it is still possible that the calcium is broken by physical therapy. We wait for two or three weeks."

I sat stunned. I did not want Ned to be operated on right before Christmas, but I had adjusted to the idea. It was very hard to change directions now. I wanted to object, to get a sense of the larger picture. What was the problem, really? Why had Dr. Waldemeyer been so sure on Monday? Why had he changed his mind now? But I knew the answer to the last question. "Chief said not to operate."

I sat silent.

"So," the surgeon went on. "Ned goes to physical therapy. He also starts swimming. I write you a recipe for the therapist on Friday. Of course, we talk before then."

Still I sat.

"Thank you for calling," I said finally. We both hung up.

Thursday was hard. Ned's class party had been rescheduled and he had to miss it because of physical therapy. Physical therapy was painful and not productive; his arm moved no more than it had in the previous two weeks. Sigrid was irritated at Dr. Waldemeyer. She thought he had moved too fast and without adequate consultation. "Ned is in physical therapy. Dr. Kolaski is the *Oberarzt* for physical therapy. Dr. Kolaski should be Ned's doctor now. He says you should not operate on someone with ninety degrees of flexion."

Ned left furious. "Dr. Waldemeyer is my doctor! I don't want another one!"

"Of course not," I said. "Sigrid does not know the situation."

"But my arm doesn't work! What's wrong with him? Why didn't he fix it?"

"He's trying, dear. It's just a bit tricky."

"It's not tricky. It's *ruined*. It will never work again! He's lying to us."

It tore my heartstrings to watch the Golux in him evaporate, his hat become describable, and the everyday world turn hard and bitter. We went for a cup of cocoa to the now familiar cafeteria of the Otto-Hoffen-Heim. Ned accepted the cocoa, but tearfully rejected my attempts at explanation and comfort. We sat and sipped; he glowered. I am but a mediocre witch and this situation required strong magic. Ned's fears were mine. In the silence I struggled to understand who and how to trust.

"I made a mistake. The lesion is on the left side of the brain."
"I am a specialist."
"Chief said not to operate."
"I made a mistake."
"Chief said not to operate."
"Ned is in out-patient physical therapy. Dr. Kolaski should be in charge of his case."

The door to the cafeteria opened and in came a doctor I recognized. He had once been in the *Gipsraum* as Ned endured some kind of cast adjustment, and he had distinguished himself by telling tales of an Australian outlaw named Ned Kelly. His curly hair and round face made him look like Grandmama's cherub. The man got himself lunch and came by our table as Ned was kicking one of its legs. "How are you?" he asked cheerfully, and then, seeing Ned's mood, he asked, "Can I help?"

"Yes," I said gratefully. "We are confused and could use a medical opinion."

Dr. Heller, so identified by his name tag, sat down at the next table. "What is the problem?" he asked Ned.

Ned would not speak, so I explained our crisis of confidence. Dr. Heller listened as he cut his meat. Then, slowly, carefully, gently, he talked to Ned, and through Ned to me. He agreed, when Ned demonstrated his range of motion, that the mobility was inadequate and should not be passively accepted. He explained that physical therapy might make the situation in Ned's elbow better and that the waiting would not make it worse. He explained that Dr. Waldemeyer was the best surgeon in northern Germany and that Ned's elbow was a particularly interesting and important problem for him. He made it clear that Dr. Waldemeyer was still Ned's doctor.

Ned listened, first silent, then asking belligerent questions, finally relaxing. "Can I have five marks for lunch?" he asked.

Dr. Heller settled down to eat his rapidly cooling lunch. His beeper went off. He made a quick phone call and came back grinning. "We're too busy," he said cheerfully. He gulped his drink and bussed the tray. "*Auf Wiedersehen!*" he called to Ned and he left. His blond curls shone and his feet melted the icy paths of the Otto-Hoffen-Heim.

Weihnachten (Christmas)

December 23, 1995

Dear Rick,

Well, all seems to be said and done for the moment—I've spent the past 24 hours shopping for Xmas. Friday was a zoo—I felt as if I were battling the whole rest of Berlin for sustenance. This morning, I went to Hertie's and got a little something for everyone. Ned went to Woolworth's with twenty marks, Brady seems to have his own plans. Now it's 2:00. Somehow, because Xmas is on Monday all the stores are closed until Wednesday. So is the Otto-Hoffen-Heim. End of issue.

One other thing, I've been putting off telling you. Last week, in response to all this, I went with Ned to get haircuts. On the spur of the moment I decided I was so gloomy and dreary that all might be improved if I just "washed away the gray!" I wanted to feel spiffy. But, it was a mistake; my hair came out kind of fire-engine red. I look like a Xmas tree ornament and clash with my new hat and scarf. Both boys are thrilled—they say I look like a swinger; Sigrid said she didn't think I was that kind of woman. I'll bring the boys with me when I pick you up at the airport tomorrow, so you don't walk past me unawares—it would be too painful.

That night the 110 bus carried the boys and me past the Otto-Hoffen-Heim, to a Christmas party at Genie's. At eight o'clock in the evening the sprawling buildings lay dark and silent. A few lights shone from a small corner of the *Hauptgebäude*—all of the patients with absolutely no alternative place to be were clustered in a single ward. It was wonderful that Ned was not among them. He nestled against me on the bus, his crooked arm forgotten. Brady sat tall and self-possessed across the aisle, torn between whether to acknowledge his connection or to be wholly independent.

At Genie's house, a warm group of people from many nations sang carols together. "*Stille Nacht, Heilige Nacht . . .*" The Americans and English tried to blend in with the Germans all around. "God rest ye merry gentlemen, let nothing you dismay . . ." A perplexed French woman asked how to parse that sentence. Brady stood suave against a wall; Ned snoozed limp on my shoulder. "Fast away the old year passes . . ." I wakened Ned for cookies and punch. Late, late in the night we took a taxi home.

Rick arrived the next morning, jet-lagged but cheery. We had brunch with the Wests. As the day wore on we chatted, listened to Christmas music, read books, and Rick slept. That evening I slept as well, until the Christmas bells awakened us. From eleven to midnight and beyond, we listened to church bells; as one stopped, another would begin. Far and near they rang and rang again. Christmas pealed into our bones.

Christmas in Berlin was very quiet and refreshingly mundane. The vagaries of Ned's medical schedule had prevented us from taking the ski vacation in the Alps we had originally seen as part of our European adventure. But just being together was enough. We had a miniscule tree, a few presents, and a little food. In fact we had very little food because somehow in the crush of the shopping I had managed to get a duck instead of a breast of goose—it is hard to stuff a family of four and a couple of guests on a duck.

During the day it snowed. It was not a dramatic snow "shaken from the sky in buckets"; it was rather a presence of snow in the air, the ground, and the trees. It transformed our suburban corner of Berlin, with its numerous wooded *Naturschutzgebieten* and little *Seen* into a sentimental postcard. Then came the cold, to maintain the effect. Day after day it held, minus-five, minus-eight, minus-ten, minus-fifteen degrees Celsius. Berlin and its many waters froze. The piece of open water at the end of the *See* shrank to nothing. For a few days the heron stood patient on the ice. Then, one morning it was gone and we did not see it again.

The city around us was, for the most part, tightly closed. Shopping expeditions had to be carefully scheduled; these trips were full-family forays as we tried to stock up for long holiday periods. Other expeditions were rare. Hockey players cleared off rinks on our little *Seen;* figure skaters shoveled serpentine paths for their use. Day after day Ned and Brady went out with their new skates on the snow-dusted ice: their wobbly first steps developed into turns and stops and going backward. Ned wore a pad on his crooked left elbow, his indescribable hat on his head. Afterward they drank cocoa from new china mugs and played chess and *Magic*.

Virtually all of the doctors were gone from the Otto-Hoffen-Heim;

the buildings stood quiet and empty, and the physical therapy department was closed for days on end. On the other days, some combination
of Ned's parents accompanied him for cheerful little sessions of elbow
moving. His arm became noticeably stronger as he worked with Sigrid
and her colleagues, but his angles did not change at all; his movement
was not spontaneously improving.

Dr. Heller had been warmly reassuring to Ned and me, but he had
shied away from discussing any issues that might lie behind the dramatic change of plan. Dr. Lyman was our next-best hope for further
information. At some point he spoke to Dr. Waldemeyer. The two
medics delighted in their exotic cross-Atlantic collaboration. Dr. Lyman
charmed Dr. Waldemeyer by opening their conversation with "*Guten
Tag*"; Dr. Waldemeyer's English sustained them past the opening. The
surgeon's grasp of the situation was impressive and Dr. Lyman's recommendation was unequivocal: "It is not a good idea to bring Ned home at
this point. It would take at least six weeks to set things in motion here,
and Dr. Waldemeyer already knows the case. He has carved Ned's
bones."

When I asked about it, the American pediatrician was unwilling to
speculate about the sudden decision not to operate. "I'm sure Dr.
Waldemeyer told you what happened. The orthopedic group voted not
to operate." Dr. Lyman did not notice that he had un-self-consciously
translated Dr. Waldemeyer's authoritarian "Professor Mahler said not to
operate" into a group action. Whatever the dynamics of the decision,
though, I suspected that his formulation was accurate and that Dr.
Waldemeyer's error in judgment was more social than physiological. I
believed his plan to operate had been overturned as much because his
colleagues were not willing to back him up for a major operation just
before Christmas as because he had been careless in his thinking about
the strength of Ned's bones.

In any case, Dr. Lyman was clear that the timing of the operation
was not crucial—it could be done equally well at any time in the next
couple of months. This seemed to give Rick and me a small window of
opportunity to take some power for ourselves. We agreed to schedule
the operation during Rick's next trip to Berlin in February. Rick left his
Christmas stay extended by a week in order to be able set up the schedule with Dr. Waldemeyer who was returning from his vacation after the
New Year.

New Year's Day fell on a Monday; on Wednesday Rick and I went to
see Dr. Waldemeyer. The doctor showed Rick the calcification in the

X rays. Rick contemplated the unmistakably cloudy areas in horror. "Shouldn't we schedule the operation as soon as possible so the calcification doesn't grow any more?"

"Yes," Dr. Waldemeyer agreed, "I always think it is best to work quickly. Mrs. Richards knows about that." He looked ruefully at me. "But I cannot schedule it until Chief comes back on January 15."

We suggested the February date; Dr. Waldemeyer looked stricken. "I have a conference in Munich that week," he said. "I have been planning it all year. There are many doctors and students there from all over Germany. I must be there." Rick and my plans were vaporized.

He consulted a calendar. "Ned comes to Station H on Monday afternoon, January 15. Chief is here then. I operate on Tuesday, January 16."

"What if Chief objects?" I asked.

"Then I do not operate. But this time Chief does not object." Dr. Waldemeyer was clear. He went on: "Ned stays here for about ten days. We move the arm in the hospital until it moves without pain. He has all his movement when he goes home from the hospital. Then he has physical therapy once or twice a week, so he remembers to move. He does not need me any more when I go to Munich."

Rick noted the dates of his February return and the two men agreed that the timing was good. Ned would be out and on vacation—we might even go skiing to keep the newly mobile arm limber. They then led the way upstairs to schedule Ned's stay with the nurses on Station H. I trailed, allowing them the comfort of planning.

Positions properly have no quantity. In an infinite, empty space every position is the same as every other. There is no way to distinguish one place from another without a point of reference from which to measure. Our notion of position is an epiphenomenon of our measuring capabilities. It is not absolute; it is not real.

That is what Newton realized over the course of years doing mathematics in his small room in Cambridge. It was a crucial insight because it allowed him to use Euclidean geometry to describe the physical world. In Euclidean geometry every place is like every other—it does not matter *where* you locate the triangles on which you are doing proofs. Newton's absolute space was Euclid's space; this meant that Newton could do mathematical physics.

Positions properly have no quantity. I could see the truth of Newton's view of space when it came to calculating planetary motions. In Berlin's Tegel airport on Friday, January 5, however, I realized that it was not adequate as an absolute. I knew that position was absolutely real and that it mattered terrifically when Rick boarded the plane and flew away.

"Are you crying, Mom? He said he's coming right back."

"Of course he is, Ned. I'm just a bit tired."

"Don't worry, Ned. Mom's fine." Brady put his arm around his brother's shoulder and smiled reassuringly at me as we walked out of the airport to the bus.

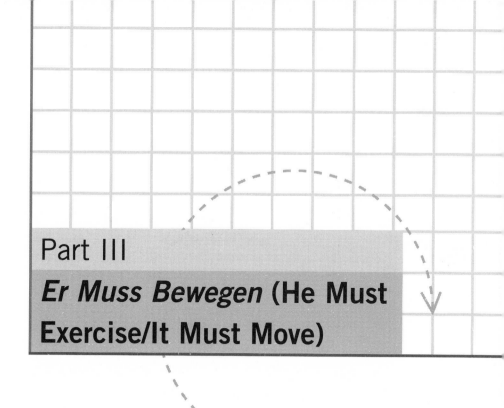

Part III

Er Muss Bewegen (He Must Exercise/It Must Move)

Dritte Operation (Third Operation)

Ned and Brady went back to school and I to my office. Physical therapy continued. Despite the seeming normality of the next week, anxieties about the impending operation hung heavily over all of our heads.

In my office De Morgan and Hamilton discussed an operation on Hamilton's daughter.

WRH to ADM, May 26, 1852

I must tell you that my daughter behaved very well yesterday—though just before the operation [for something near her eye], she whispered to me that she *should* like to be put asleep. She had been given her choice. You would have mesmerized her; I was content with chloroform, and the dose given was not enough to prevent her from having a sort of dreamlike consciousness. She is doing very well. My cousin Hutton is a skilful surgeon.

ADM to WRH May 27, 1852

I am very glad your daughter is out of it, I hope for good and all. Where chloroform can be ventured upon, it is more speedy than mesmerism [a nineteenth-century form of hypnosis], which requires some previous trials. There is a kind of consciousness left by both, very often. The first man operated upon (amputation of the leg) by mesmerism in England said "he felt a *crunching*"—it was the *saw!*—"but it did not hurt."

I do not have great faith in hypnotism as an approach to anesthetics, so I was glad that it was Hamilton's daughter and not Alice who was operated on. I was also glad that the little girl did so well. But clarity on these issues did not resolve my anxieties. Hamilton's daughter was not Ned, and the outcome of his operation was still unknown.

I struggled to come to grips with Dr. Waldemeyer's meaning when he said: *"The child will have a lot of pain."* Neither the doctor nor I had any trouble knowing the meaning of the words in this sentence, but as I turned it over in my mind I realized how loaded it was. I did not know what Ned's decisive young surgeon thought of when he thought of a child, and I was equally unsure of what his definition of pain might be. All of the discussion about the catheter, whether implanting it was a procedure that could be done to a child, contributed to my anxieties. I was worried about what we were getting Ned into.

In the New Year's appointment I had let Rick and the doctor do the planning, and they had reserved a bed for Ned on the ward. The rationale was the same as mine had been in early December; they thought it would be better for Ned to have peer companionship than to be isolated in a private room. When Dr. Waldemeyer presented this decision to the nurses on Station H, however, it seemed to me that their reaction was ambivalent at best. So, in a preoperative phone call with Dr. Waldemeyer, I reopened the question of whether Ned should be in a room where I could stay with him.

"If it were your child," I began, using a formula Dr. Lyman had given me as a way to ask a doctor for advice, "would you put Ned into a private room?"

There was a silence and I wondered what I had done. Then, as if he had made a major decision, Dr. Waldemeyer responded to my question. "I have two children," he said. "The older one is almost thirteen." His voice dripped with loving pride. "She has a birthday just next week! For her I do not think my wife would stay. She likes to be independent and would work well with the nurses. My other child is younger," he went on, in a warmly humorous key, "like Ned. He can be frightened. For him I think my wife would stay."

It was my turn to pause. In German there is a sharp distinction between formal interactions in which *you* is translated as *Sie* and intimate ones in which *you* is translated as *du*. It is notoriously hard for English speakers to figure out the boundaries between the two; we struggled with them constantly in *Gruppe B*. I knew that all conversations between doctor and patient would be in the *Sie* form. But my question was formulated in a language and a culture where the distinction between formal and personal interactions is blurred and linguistically unmarked. In Dr. Waldemeyer's pause I heard his attempt to deal with the *Sie/du* problem in reverse; to navigate unexpected shoals that would have been clearly marked had we been speaking his language. To a German, it seemed, my hypothetical question was considerably stronger than I had intended, and pushed into personal space. It caught him off guard, but he responded by letting me in. I was touched and, accepting the analogy between our sons, I asked him to switch Ned to a private room.

❀ ❀ ❀

Putting Ned into a private room meant that I had to move in with him. Brady was happy with this arrangement. His thirst for independence was strong and he was intrigued by a life in which he could collect leftovers from the meals at the *Wissenschaftskolleg* and eat them in the apartment, when and as he liked. Coming to the Otto-Hoffen-Heim on his way home from school seemed enough parental control to him and, after some thought, to me as well. We agreed that he would take on the job of daily e-mail communication with Rick when I could not make it to my office.

So, on the morning of Monday the fifteenth, Ned and I packed books, CDs, and clothes for both night and day, and schlepped them to the Otto-Hoffen-Heim on the 110 bus. We went first for physical therapy and moral support to Sigrid where Ned showed off the large Steif panther Matteus's family had contributed to ease hospital fears. *Schnell,* Fast, was the animal's name. Ned set him on a filing cabinet, but his gleaming green eyes so startled the other patients that I had to bring the animal down and hide him under a coat on my lap.

After Ned and Sigrid had gone through their paces, and the assorted physical therapists had wished Ned luck, he and I carted our belongings to Station H. Schnell and Racky watched us from the pillow as we unpacked into *Zimmer Acht,* the same private room we had occupied during October's *Notfall.* It felt like a major move. The first operation had been so sudden that my center of gravity had never really shifted, and with the second, I was always a force outside of the system pulling to free Ned of its entanglements. But this time both Ned and I really moved into the hospital.

The preoperative process on Tuesday morning proceeded in fits and starts, seemingly always planned to take place when I was not there. The nurses had said that Ned was to be the second operation of the day, probably leaving between nine-thirty and ten. So, at about seven-thirty I left him calmly in the room as I slipped out for a quick breakfast. When I returned at about eight, he was fearful and alone.

"Where were you, Mom? They shaved my arm and you weren't here!"

"Already? I'm sorry, Ned. I was at breakfast, where I said I'd be. I'm right here now and I won't go anywhere."

"Is Liza coming soon?" Genie was out of town but Liza had volunteered to be with me through the operation. She had promised Ned she would be there before the operation so he could talk to her.

"At about nine. For now, let me read you a chapter."

✿ ✿ ✿

"Is Liza coming, Mom?" It was getting close to nine.

"Yes, she should be here soon. Maybe I should check to make sure she knows where we are."

I went out to look for Liza but didn't see her. When I returned, no more than five minutes later, Ned's bed was in the hall about to be wheeled over to the operating theater. He had drunk his sedative but was nonetheless panicked. Things were moving faster than either of us had expected.

They continued to do so. I learned how patients were transported during cold weather as the nurses sprinted with Ned and his bed to the operating theater. I ran alongside and held his hand until they whisked him unceremoniously through the doors where I could not go. As I turned away, Liza came briskly up the path, books under her arm, fox-tail hat on her head. She had planned her arrival carefully so she would have time to chat with Ned before he was taken away; as it was, she missed him entirely.

Getting Ned into the operating theater was quick; getting him out again was not. Time crawled. All afternoon I sat by the hot drinks machine facing the path to the operating theater. People wandered in and out, buying coffee, chatting with their children, bundling up for expeditions outdoors. I sat and looked at them, or the path, or, determinedly, at my book.

Finally at about four o'clock, two racing nurses pelted through the cold with Ned's bed; simultaneously Dr. Waldemeyer appeared from his office on my right. "The operation was good!" he told me as Ned and his nurses disappeared into the elevator. I indicated that I wanted to follow but the doctor was too involved to let me go. "I removed the calcification," he explained, "but that was not enough. So I had to open the capsule from both sides to loosen it. He has two scars now but the movement should be much better." The female doctor with the long blond hair appeared and Dr. Waldemeyer raised his voice to include her in his triumphant announcement: "We got 10 degrees of extension and 140 degrees of flexion," he crowed. She smiled happily at him as we went up the stairs together.

The two doctors peeled off into the ward as I hurried to *Zimmer Acht*. Ned was there, looking small and weak but alert. Two blood bags, one from each of the incisions, hung from his splinted arm. In his armpit, above the splint, a couple of wires curled out and then in again; close by was a shunt through which the anesthetic could be delivered to the catheter hidden somewhere deep in his arm. The catheter did not hurt him but putting it in had been a frightening experience. But now it was past, and after a brief complaint Ned settled down.

Soon Dr. Waldemeyer arrived, accompanied by a few of his followers.

"It goes well, and now you have two scars!" he said cheerily to Ned as he unwrapped the bandage.

"No, I have three," Ned drowsily clarified. "I have one on my head too."

The surgeon grinned, and then gently began to move the arm. Like a door on its hinge it moved effortlessly back and forth. With each pass blood oozed into one or another of the bags, but since Ned felt nothing at all it somehow was not troublesome. I got a momentary glimpse of the surgical perspective that can work on limbs without a thought to the person to whom they are attached.

As he moved it, Dr. Waldemeyer explained the program for the next few days. Ned's arm was to be moved as much as possible. Between times, it was to be placed into one of two casts; one bent to about 110 degrees of flexion, the other extended to 10 degrees. The basic instruction was that the casts were to be changed every four hours, night and day, but he overruled this for the first night so that Ned could sleep. For the time being, then, Ned would be in the bending cast; the extension one lay on the desk.

The next day was the beginning of the rest of Ned's life as it was to be at the Otto-Hoffen-Heim. Dr. Waldemeyer arrived early in the morning and introduced us to Petra, Ned's physical therapist. She was a sprightly young woman with a short thatch of unabashedly dyed red hair. She was very young, closer to twenty than twenty-five. It was her first week on the job. Ned took to her immediately.

Petra sat by Ned's side and moved his arm up and down while a machine slowly, constantly, measured anesthetic into the catheter. She chatted with Ned and we all watched the Australian Open on the television. It was the perfect entertainment, as it was not particularly frenetic and essentially linguistically transparent; the sound on the set did not work well in any case, so we simply turned it off. We all watched Boris Becker take on a hapless Swede, and Ned wept for the loser as Petra moved his arm up and down on its hinge.

At noon, having spent several half-hour sessions with Ned, Petra explained that she would be back after lunch. Ned was asleep when she returned, and we agreed that it was best not to disturb him. Wednesday was a half day for her, but I had seen what she had done and was completely confident that I could do it as well. Dr. Waldemeyer had said he would stop by before a four o'clock lecture. If there were any problems I could check with him.

Ned was awake by about two-thirty. Refreshed by our naps we turned the TV back on—the available fare was a repeat of the match we had seen that morning. I unwrapped Ned's arm from the protective splint and sat down in Petra's chair by his side. Eyes on the Australian open, I slowly moved the arm towards Ned's shoulder. Blood began to ooze into one of the bags. Ned flinched and yelped. I stopped, startled. After a brief pause I tried again only to meet the same resistance.

"Don't do that! It hurts! " he told me.

I backed off, perplexed. The anesthetic syringe was not yet empty and the machine delivering Ned his measured dose seemed to be operating properly; Ned was in the same position he had been in the morning, and I was doing precisely what I had seen Petra doing.

Gently I tried again only to meet with the same protest. "Don't do that! It hurts!" he wailed.

"What if we warm it up slowly," I suggested. "Let's just move it a little and try to move it more when you have loosened up bit."

Tearfully, Ned agreed, and I moved it in a much restricted arc. Things were fine as long as I did not push his limits, but they were narrow and did not seem to broaden over time. In fact I began to fear they were shrinking. Ned and I entered into an ever-more-complex set of negotiations of a kind known best, if not only, to parents of preadolescents. By the end of half an hour I set forth down the dark corridor to consult with a nurse. She said simply that she was not a physical therapist and did not know about it. I returned to Ned's bedside, gently moved his arm through a tiny arc, and waited for Dr. Waldemeyer.

At about four-thirty, Dr. Heller came in to change the anesthetic syringe. He was there to perform a mechanical process and had little to offer about Ned's arm and its pain. When I asked him about the problem of moving the elbow, he suggested that I lay off for a while, that Ned's stress might be counterproductive to the process. I took his point and retired to the couch. But then I began to worry that Ned's arm was not even bent enough to fit into the cast he was supposed to wear for the night, and returned to the fray. I was right to be concerned. Ned's arm had lost a great deal of flexion during the two hours that I had been feebly moving it in ever-decreasing arcs. It was a painful, confrontational process to put it back into its bending cast; Ned cried and protested but I refused to back off. We were both exhausted when the deed was finally done.

Again ensconced on the couch I watched Ned watching TV. I could almost see the angry tangle of confusion and remembered pain hanging in a comic-book bubble over his head. Mine was similarly dark and matted. I focused on the little wires that curled in and out of his arm and followed my thoughts to the brief aside about pain that I'd noticed in Hamilton's and De Morgan's usually mathematical correspondence. What made the piece interesting was not that they were debating whether it was better to use chemistry or mesmerism for anesthesia but that the interchange began with the question of whether it was a good idea to use anesthesia at all. The two men were writing within a decade of the first surgical success with anesthesia. Until then, pain was a character issue, to be borne with a stiff upper lip.

But in the Otto-Hoffen-Heim the doctors were in charge of Ned's pain; I needed Dr. Waldemeyer. He had obviously gone to his lecture, but five-fifteen seemed like a reasonable time to begin looking for him to come by. When five-forty-five went by with no sign I went to the nurses' station and asked where he might be. The nurses said that if he had said he would come, he would. I readjusted my calculations on the basis of a two-hour lecture. By six-fifteen, however, I returned, impatient, to the nurses' station. I explained my concern to a gently competent one with long black hair, who seemed to be in charge for the evening; she called Dr. Waldemeyer's beeper and reported cheerfully that it was on, which was a good sign. I returned to Ned's side to wait. At seven-thirty I again ventured forth to ask where Dr. Waldemeyer might be. The dark-haired nurse seemed perplexed, as she said she did not know and called his beeper again. Again, she assured me, it had beeped, which was to the good. Again I returned to Ned's bedside to wait.

By eight-fifteen I had had enough. I was in a hospital and ultimately it was someone else's job to care for my son. I went back to the nurses' station.

"Ned has to be put in his extending cast," I said. "I can't do it. I need your help."

"OK," the nurse said. "I come when I can."

Fifteen minutes later she arrived and for fifteen minutes we worked on the problem. We breathed with Ned, we exhorted him to relax, we pulled on his arm—all to no avail. The pain was excruciating and neither of us had the necessary force—psychological or physical—to effect the change. Finally the nurse recognized the reality of the problem I had been struggling with alone for the afternoon. She went down the hall to call an anesthesiologist. The one who arrived fifteen minutes later was the warm, cheerful man who before Christmas had witnessed my bloody nose. He quickly and expertly went to work, first with an injection to stop the pain. He then checked the wires that led in and out of Ned's arm, fiddled with the shunt, and adjusted the machine and syringe. As he worked, he explained what he was trying to do.

"Is this hot or cold?" he asked Ned as he rested a cup of hot water on his arm. When Ned was not sure, the doctor beamed. "The first thing to go is the hot or cold feeling," he said, "second goes pain, third goes moving the muscles. We want the middle, movement with no pain. I come back in an hour and see how you are doing!" he reassured Ned as he went out the door.

It was already well past Ned's bedtime, but he and I waited calmly for the return of the anesthesiologist. True to his word the doctor came back at ten and tested to see that the arm was truly painless. It was not only painless but also limp and lifeless.

"That's fine," he assured Ned. "You don't need to move it when you sleep."

Ned slept well, but I did not. I was furious. It was not just the specific evening but the whole situation that was so infuriating: I resented needing Dr. Waldemeyer so much.

I knew what I wanted to say, but I was less clear about how to say it. I did not want to confront the doctor in front of Ned; any disagreement between us was very upsetting for him. I was also unwilling to dress the doctor down in front of the cast of characters who usually accompanied him. Their witnessing might imbue my criticism with other issues in ways I did not know. I was angry but I did not want to cause undue trouble. I plotted ways to talk to him alone.

I need not have bothered; Dr. Waldemeyer had no intention of talking to me alone. By the time he showed himself to me at about eight-thirty on Thursday morning, he had been totally apprised of what had happened the preceding evening and had the situation well in hand. He arrived accompanied by Petra as well as his supporting medical staff, to give Ned an anesthetic drip as well as changing the syringe.

"I don't want him to be in pain," he explained.

"Fine," I said, "but what am I to do if he *is* in pain?"

"Call me," he said. "The nurses know how to reach me."

"But I tried," I retorted. "We called you two times last night and you never called back."

"I did not get back from my lecture until after ten," he said "and then I was very tired and Ned was asleep."

"I don't care where you were," I insisted. "You weren't there when the nurses called and I could not get the help I needed."

Dr. Waldemeyer's entourage seemed a bit startled, and he blinked. Then he explained the on-call system of the hospital staff and assured me that if we called the doctor in charge, someone would always come within an hour. I thanked him as I made a note of what to do in the future.

Zimmer Acht (Room Eight)

Surrounded by Station H, *Zimmer Acht* was splendidly isolated. It became more so as the week progressed: When Ned and I first arrived we could use the telephone, within the first day we lost the ability to call out, by the second no one could call in. On the third day, after swallowing several of my coins at random, the public phone downstairs went out too. From then on Ned and I were totally dependent on actual visitors for communication. In this we were blessed. Brady was a faithful presence, keeping watch over his brother and mother every day after school. He also maintained communication by phone and e-mail to Rick, far away in Providence.

We had other visitors as well. From the *Wissenschaftskolleg* came mothers of children, Beth and Helge. The rector contributed his son's prized Gameboy, and the *Verwaltung* sent a stuffed hedgehog who nestled by Ned's pillow. From the Max Planck Institute came everyone. Plato came with books for me and a Leggo set for Ned. Snorri came with more books and a wealth of Icelandic perspectives. Clare came with a swirl of fur and a box of candy. Liza came and engaged Ned in lively conversation. Genie and her daughter came, bearing fruit, cheese, and a set of Garrison Keillor tapes. They coordinated their visits so we would be covered but not overwhelmed. They warmed and enlivened *Zimmer Acht,* turning it into a cozy home for Ned and me.

Petra became an ever-more-welcome addition to our lives. With me she was at first somewhat shy and deferential, but with Ned she was magic. She unflinchingly accepted his view of himself as a swinging American teenager and cheerfully entertained his interpretations of the world. "R.E.M. is the coolest group. Except for the Grateful Dead. Do you know the Grateful Dead?" Initially I had some illusions about her teaching him German, but neither of them was interested in anything so drearily didactic. Instead he taught her ever more subtle turns of American phrase and explained remembered puns of Rick's. She taught him phrases of Bavarian dialect and told him about her childhood in a tiny German town. Through it all she moved his arm: "Bend . . . stretch . . . bend . . . and stretch. Good, Ned! Now let it loose."

I am sure that life at the *Wissenschaftskolleg* continued from January 16 to 22, but I was watching the Australian Open Tennis Tournament. At times it seemed that the whole event was being staged for our particular benefit. The people in *Zimmer Acht* were constantly engaged in long contemplations on the players' attire, the different languages in which they were probably thinking, various styles and strategies of play, what they did with the second ball when serving with the first. We rooted for different people, basing our choices on a host of odd criteria: their facial expressions, tempers, hair length, or color of headbands. Important matches, with stars like Bjorn Borg, André Agassi, or Monica Seles, were often repeated; we found ourselves drawn into various dramas again and again, trying to change our allegiances to avoid weeping a second time over the loss of a favorite, to analyze the moment at which a match with a known outcome turned.

I remember one particularly crowded moment with assorted people from the Max Planck Institute on the couch and a smattering of medical personnel in attendance. The TV was on but silently, and the air buzzed with various conversations. Petra was moving Ned's arm while Dr. Waldemeyer watched and talked to his followers. No one was paying much attention to Ned himself. Suddenly he squealed, flinging his right arm up with such force that his whole body levitated. The room froze; Dr. Waldemeyer tensed and jerked to attention. Slowly the roomful of adults realized that what Ned had said was "Yes!!" and that it was directed to the television screen. Palpable relief spread over the doctor's face. He grinned ruefully and shook his head.

In the nights *Zimmer Acht* was as permeable as it was during the day. We were always liable to be interrupted by medical arrivals or the alarm of Ned's anesthetic running low. Grandmama neglected to provide me with protocols for how to act when strangers materialize in your bedroom. Sometimes I opened my eyes, sometimes I didn't, unsure which stance gave the greater illusion of dignity. The passive approach seemed to work well. It also allowed the possibility of eavesdropping, and overheard nighttime conversations could be useful to my attempts to figure out the ins and outs of life on Station H.

One night I overheard a female anesthesiologist ask the nurse about chocolate stains on Ned's cover.

"The cover is dirty," the doctor said. "It has to be changed."

"I know," the nurse replied. "It has been that way for the past two days. I wonder when she will change it."

They left clicking their tongues at my low standards.

It had never occurred to me that I would be held responsible for changing Ned's linens. But over time I realized that Ned's cleanliness in general was my responsibility. As the week wore on, he began to be given enough time between syringe changes to take brief walks and use the toilet. If the gap stretched into a long period, I sometimes performed the acrobatic task of bathing him with all due respect to the water-soluble splint and vulnerable shunt in his upper arm. The nurses contributed nothing, not even soap.

Sunday was a particularly difficult time for physical therapy. There was only one half-day physical therapist for the entire hospital, but Dr. Waldemeyer had insisted that Ned have two sessions by being both the first and last patient. It was a far cry from the weekday's four or even five sessions, but it was better than nothing.

At six that Sunday morning, Ned's syringe ran out. I alerted the nurses and we waited, but no doctor appeared. I took advantage of Ned's freedom from the catheter to give him a much-needed bath. Even after this elaborate procedure was completed and Ned was clean from top to bottom, there was no sign of a doctor to renew Ned's syringe. I reminded the nurses but they said they could do nothing. Seven o'clock moved toward seven-thirty. The physical therapist was to come at eight. Frustrated, I decided to take matters into my own hands and tried to generate action in the only way I could think of: I put on my coat, my hat, and my mittens and ventured into the frigid darkness to the telephones in the basement of the *Hauptgebäude*, the main building.

"Guten tag. Sie haben die Nummer 555 31 18 in Berlin gewählt. Hinterlassen Sie bitte eine Nachricht. Ich rufe Sie bald möglich zurück. Vielen Dank."

"Hello, Dr. Waldemeyer. This is Joan Richards, Ned's mother, calling from the hospital at seven-thirty on Sunday morning. I am calling because you have made it clear that it is crucially important that Ned have physical therapy two times today. But his syringe has not been changed in the past hour and a half, and if it is not done soon, he will not be anesthetized for his eight o'clock physical therapy. The situation may be resolved by the time you get this message, but I do not know any other way to get things done in this hospital. Thank you."

When I got back to Ned's room the syringe still had not been renewed. Irritated, I asked the nurses what I could do.

"We have just called the doctor again. He is coming right away."

I was glad to hear he was on his way, but I was not totally convinced. "What can I do if he doesn't come?" I asked.

"*Schimpfen Sie mit ihm!*" the nurse responded cheerfully.

Schimpfen—it was a word that I had recently memorized as I worked my way through a vocabulary book purporting to be a list of the 2,000 most common German words. It means "to chew out; to curse," what Ned would call "to yell at." It suddenly struck me that this was what Big Nurz had done to me when I first arrived on Station H.

The physical therapist arrived at about eight o'clock, but the nurses had to turn her away because Ned's arm was not anesthetized. She promised to try again at nine. At about eight-fifteen, a young, sleepy doctor arrived. The nurses congregated hopefully as the doctor and I faced each other.

"Where in the world have you been?" I began, trying to sound appropriately fierce. "Ned has been without anesthetic for more than two hours now! We had to turn the physical therapist away."

"There was an emergency last night," the young man replied. "I did not get to sleep until five o'clock and the *Oberarzt* decided to let me sleep."

"I can understand that you are tired, but Ned's elbow doesn't make this kind of distinction," I said. "It needs to be tended whether you are tired or not."

"Well, let me do it then," he replied and turned his attention to the syringe. The nurses left disappointed; in comparison to Big Nurz I was a total wimp.

About five minutes later my call to Dr. Waldemeyer bore fruit in the form of a call for me at the nurses station.

"Has Ned's syringe been changed yet?" the doctor asked.

"Yes," I said. "A young man just did it. But the basic situation is really bad. The nurses can't get the doctors to do things when they ask."

"Well," Dr. Waldemeyer answered. "I just made a call over there and I . . . I don't know how to say in English but '*Ich habe mit ihnen geschimpft.*' They do not let it go so long again."

Almost before I had a chance to hang up, the young doctor returned to give Ned an extra anesthetic injection, confirm that the physical therapist would soon reappear, and apologize for having not changed the syringe more promptly.

If the fine art of *schimpfen* defined a cultural divide between me and Station H, the issue of names did even more so. Very few of the medical personnel wore name tags, and they never introduced themselves. By the end of a couple of days in which *Zimmer Acht* was constantly invaded by anonymous strangers, the problem of introductions became a cause célèbre. I confided my frustration to Petra and she was wickedly delighted that I noticed. "We learned in school that it is important for patients to know our names. But the nurses and doctors never listen to us."

I asked what would be the most polite way for me to ask.

"You could try '*Wurden Sie sich mir bitte vorstellen?*' [roughly 'Would you please introduce yourself to me?'] It is very polite, but I still don't think they would like it."

The next time a couple of doctors came to check on Ned's syringe, Petra twinkled expectantly at me. But the young men were so distant and self-contained I did not have what it took to use her line.

"Chicken!" Ned teased after they had left.

I came to see the complete lack of introductions as the other side of the coin of my total dependence on Dr. Waldemeyer. In this system, he and he alone was Ned's doctor. All of the other people were no more than functionaries in a big machine that Dr. Waldemeyer coordinated.

Der Katheter (The Catheter)

Monday, January 22

Ned was doing fine; his arm was moving well. Since I felt I needed to return to the Villa Walther I moved him out of *Zimmer Acht* and onto same bed in *Zimmer Eins* he had occupied before Christmas. I stayed by his bed to help him settle in, but at the end of the day I left.

It was an infinite relief to be home again, or whatever the proper name would be for our apartment. The first thing I did was to call Rick. We talked about our son, how tough and resilient, how sharp and funny, how basically wonderful he was. He was still in the middle of a process, but we agreed that it was going well. The whole situation seemed good and clear.

When I hung up I had dinner with Brady. After a week on his own, even my independent sixteen-year-old was glad for some company. We talked about his plans for the upcoming term: ". . . and Mom? Since I've already had it, I decided to sign up for physics in German." He was growing wonderfully into his new environment. It was fun to be with him.

After dinner Brady settled into his homework and I made some phone calls. With Ned on the ward I figured I would have middays free, and it was high time to get back to work. I set up a couple of meetings with people I'd been putting off for months. I invited Rudolf to lunch at the *Kolleg* in hopes he could ease me back into thinking about my Victorians. Then I arranged to meet Genie for breakfast in the hospital cafeteria on Thursday, so she could say "Hi" to Ned afterward. I was glad to be getting back on track.

Tuesday, January 23

The next day marked the beginning of a commuting schedule. It began in the pitch dark at about five-forty-five, when I walked the two blocks to my office to receive and send e-mail. When I got back at about six-fifteen, I woke Brady and we coordinated our days while he ate his cornflakes.

Then, somewhere between six-forty-five and seven, I set off for the Otto-Hoffen-Heim. If I walked briskly it took just over an hour for me to get from the Villa Walther to the hospital. The route I chose lay through the Grunewald—I liked the peace of the night trees. There was little fear of crime in my area of Berlin; in any case a combination of the bitter cold and the ubiquitous dogs, always accompanied by their owners, would have discouraged even the most determined human menace. As I strode down the straight, dark paths toward my son my legs would tingle with the cold and my soul would untangle.

This Tuesday morning I arrived to find Ned in a snit. The previous evening, after I had left him defenseless, he had fought with a nurse who insisted that the new Polartec pajamas Rick had brought for Christmas were day clothes and made him sleep in underpants and a T-shirt. In response, Ned refused to wear his pajamas in the day. When I arrived they were at a standoff and he was bare-chested under the covers. I firmly put his wrinkly T-shirt back on and set out to buy undeniably German *Schlafanzug*, pajamas.

It being Tuesday, my shopping expedition had to be wrapped around the *Wissenschaftskolleg*'s seminar and formal lunch. There I listened intently to a lecture about Goethe. My question was about what the German writer/scientist thought of Newtonian space. At lunch I sat at the speaker's table, anxious to pursue my interest further. "You asked a good question," he said. "I didn't think you could understand so much of the talks! Your German is getting better and better. What kinds of things do you do in German class?" He had no intention of discussing Goethe with an American woman. Still, as I rode the bus up the Kurfürsten-damm to buy Ned's new clothes, I entertained myself with thoughts about different views of space, and the ways we move between them.

By about four o'clock, when I got back to the Otto-Hoffen-Heim with my sartorial offerings, Ned seemed to be facing a more substantive medical problem. His catheter was beginning to wear out, as everyone knew it would. Ned was becoming uncomfortable even when it was delivering the anesthetic: he could feel hot and cold on his arm and it was beginning to ache. I mentioned this to Dr. Waldemeyer as he raced from one place to another.

I could see why the doctor did not want to take up the question of Ned's anesthetic at five in the afternoon. Ned had no more physical therapy scheduled for the day and had a cast that kept his arm still and basically painless. I also decided to let the matter ride until the next day since Wednesday mornings seemed to be grand rounds. At that time I assumed I could find out whatever new anesthetic regime was being put into place.

Wednesday, January 24

I was so anxious not to miss the rounds that I arrived at eight-fifteen, before visiting hours. There were no doctors in evidence, but Ned was in need of one. He lay on his bed, reduced by a pain that he dated to the midnight change of the anesthetic syringe. Since then his elbow had hurt so relentlessly he had not been able to sleep. When I arrived, he had not been able to move enough either to wash or to eat his breakfast. The TV's constant noise was bothering him. He was in a bad way.

I washed Ned's face, and then I went out to talk to the nurses. They were aware of the problem. So was Petra who was huddled in the hall with the other physical therapists wondering how she was to exercise his arm. Neither of these groups had the power to take any action with respect to the catheter, though. I asked whether a doctor was coming and Petra said "I hope so." It was hardly an encouraging statement, but not one I took terribly seriously. Ned was, after all, in a hospital, and his problem was one that had been predicted long before.

Besides, on this particular morning, my other child needed me. There were things that Brady was not ready to deal with alone and one of them was particularly pressing. He had broken his glasses. Without them he could not see well enough to make school attendance meaningful. That afternoon he had a variety of activities that he did not want to cancel because of blindness. I left Ned's bedside to pursue a pair of backup glasses for his brother.

I worked with dispatch, however, and by ten-fifteen was back at Ned's bedside. He was in the same condition—pale and in pain, diminished in his bed. I went out in search of the intern on the floor in hopes that he was in a better position to help than were the nurses. He came to Ned's bed and gazed at the miserable child. "I know," he said. "I've called over twice, but they have not sent anyone yet. I am only an intern. I don't want to get a bad reputation. I cannot call again."

No doctor arrived, but Petra did. I had a luncheon appointment so I left her and Ned to their linguistic adventures. But when I got to the *Wissenschaftskolleg* I just apologized to the woman I was to meet and took the bus back. It was by then twelve-thirty. Ned's condition was unchanged except that someone had renewed the anesthetic syringe. I knew that this had to have been done by a doctor—one had been on the scene but had apparently done nothing about the central problem. I sat by Ned's bed and read to him while I tried to work out my next move.

The black-haired nurse arrived with some pills for Ned.

"What are those?" I asked.

"Tylenol," she answered.

"What for?" I asked.

"To bring down his fever," she replied.

I panicked. I had known that the defunct catheter was hurting Ned, but that it was infecting him as well did not occur to me until that moment. It marked the end of my attempt to be reasonable, nondemanding, and trusting. I flew down the stairs to find a doctor. I was ready to tackle any white-suited person who crossed my path and to dismantle the stuccoed walls of the Otto-Hoffen-Heim piece by piece until one did.

In the event, such drastic measures were unnecessary. Dr. Waldemeyer was in his office downstairs. It was the end of a busy day with patients; perhaps the early morning surgery had pushed them into an even greater concentration. I gnashed my teeth in a line outside the door to the doctor's office while he talked on the phone and his secretary handled various routine requests. Finally it was my turn, and I explained the problem in my choppy German: "My son is not well. The catheter does not work any more. His arm is very painful. He has a fever. He needs Dr. Waldemeyer immediately."

The secretary dutifully wrote the message while Dr. Waldemeyer smiled at me through his conversation. I refrained from spitting in my rage and raced back upstairs. There I found Ned with Petra, beaming. "Surprise!" he crowed. "They took out the catheter!" Sure enough, the wires were gone from his arm, the machine from his bedside. Already Ned felt better and Petra was more comfortable moving his arm. There were broad smiles all around and they went back to work: I left them to it and paced the hall.

Dr. Waldemeyer appeared, breathless. "I got your message," he said. "How is he now?"

I explained about the catheter and the pain. "Why don't you tell me sooner?" he asked as he quickly took charge. "We give him something to stop the pain immediately. It makes him to sleep but I want him to forget the pain. I want him not to be afraid. I want him to move his arm."

"What about the fever?" I asked.

Dr. Waldemeyer looked stricken. "That is not good," he said and ran to the nurses station. Soon thereafter he ran back: "Everything is in order, now," he said. "The nurses and the other doctors take care of everything. I am out of town for two days," he went on. "Dr. Kawalek is in charge of Ned." My horror at the thought of a strange doctor in charge at this point must have been clear on my face. "Don't worry," Dr.

Waldemeyer said genially, before he hurried away. "He is *Oberarzt*, like me. He takes good care of Ned."

The doctor was gone, but within minutes his effect was evident. A bevy of medics gathered around Ned, giving him injections, taking blood, and hooking up his IV. I danced around the action, unwilling to leave but not wanting to be in the way. The unknown Dr. Kawalek was on my mind—I had no idea who he was. In a momentary lull I asked the intern, hoping for a description that might help me to place him among all of the nameless doctors I had come across in the last few months.

"Dr. Kawalek? *Aja!* Don't worry. He is *Oberarzt*, like Waldemeyer." Apparently once I knew Dr. Kawalek's position, I knew everything there was to know. Knowing what he looked like, whether I had ever spoken to him before, what kind of man he was, was totally irrelevant. By this time, I had been around long enough to recognize that since an *Oberarzt* had power it was important that one had Ned in his sights. I tried to let that be enough.

Within fifteen minutes Ned was comfortable and serene. Brady arrived, having canceled his after-school plans because he was worried. The brothers settled down cozily together, and I left to calm myself with a turn around the *Naturschutzgebiet*. My nose and eyes ran as I walked a figure eight through the woods.

At first I thought of people skating for miles on the frozen expanses, up and down Berlin's rivers. I mourned for my feisty Ned, always so eager, determined, and strong. I wanted to seize the moment in this special time and place; I wanted to skate with him around the *Pfaueninsel*. As I walked along, the frigid trees began to calm me. I began the second loop deeper in the small woods, thinking about the wild birds my newspaper told me were flocking to the zoo in search of unfrozen water. I thought about the heron long vanished from our *See*, and wondered whether he was among them. I wondered how the fox was doing in the face of such cold—about dens, fur, and hibernation.

Suddenly I came across a pile of feathers in the path. The fox was nowhere to be seen but the plight of this bird was evidence that somehow she was surviving. But I was not comforted. I was frightened. Ned, my *federnd*, resilient little boy, seemed to have more in common with the bird than with its predator. I almost ran out of the woods.

When I arrived at Ned's side I found that I had missed some action. Soon after I had left, his IV had fallen out, dripping his medicaments onto the bed. Brady had responded quickly and effectively, and by the time I reappeared the sheets had been changed and the paraphernalia removed. There was little room for this kind of confusion in the ordered world of my adolescent mathematician, though; as soon as I arrived, Brady remembered a physics test and fled.

As he was leaving, the long-blond-haired doctor was bustling about preparing an injection as an alternative to the drip. The shot was going into Ned's buttock; he chose to have it standing up between the doctor and me but was not at all relaxed about it. He stood between the two of us, trembling with nerves and fever. It seemed a good moment for friendly calming banter between mother and doctor, a time to help Ned forget himself by giving him something else to relate to. As a way to start, it seemed genial to exchange names with this woman who was, in fact, the first doctor Ned and I had encountered in our odyssey through the Otto-Hoffen-Heim.

"Würden Sie sich mir bitte vorstellen?" I addressed her over Ned's head, which was buried in my breast.

"Sie wissen wie ich heisse," she retorted sharply. "You know my name! I have worked with Ned since the first operation!"

"Ja!" I replied, trying to stay light. "I know you have. But I do not know your name."

My attempt at friendliness failed. The situation was fraught with tension, and my question provided a focus for the young woman's irritations. *"Ich heisse von Lennert,"* she hissed. *"Dr. von Lennert."* Her voice rose as she warmed to her topic. "I spell it for you if you need! V-O-N, Von, L-E-N-N-E-R-T, Lennert." She fairly spat the letters at me as I cradled Ned's head. *"Frau Dr. von Lennert,"* she went on. "Would you like me to write it down?"

"No thank you," I said. "I'll not forget."

It was not the response I had expected or hoped for, but it did have the effect of taking Ned's mind off of the shot the doctor delivered to his buttock. He climbed back onto the bed and she left. The various injections began to take effect, and Ned went to sleep. Alone and thoroughly *geschimpft,* I sat beside my son's bed on Station H as twilight deepened into night.

A tiny snippet of poetry appeared unbidden, and floated around my head:

'Tis all in pieces, all coherence gone;
All just supply and all relation.

I did not know where it came from, but it fit.

Ned was still in a deep sleep when the end of parental visiting hours meant I had to leave. I set out on foot for the Villa Walther, hoping for calm in exercise. I did not venture into the Grunewald. Its straight paths bespoke an order that excluded me and mine, and its evening darkness threatened in a way the morning did not. I walked down the Clayallee, past a sad, drunken huddle of American ex-soldiers and down the road between the deserted barracks and the embassy. A tank hulked menacingly on the barracks side—part of some leftover celebration of American might. The embassy was surrounded by fences and barbed wire. I found no comfort in being American.

I walked toward the residential section of the Grunewald. Passing cars caught me in their lights; deep in their dark interiors there were people thinking thoughts in German as they drove through their city. Many of the street signs were double; in addition to the current names they sported small notices of their former ones—Jewish names that had been erased in the Nazi period. At crossings, lights flashed their signals. I followed their directions carefully, even when there was no one to note or appreciate my cooperation. When I paused to respect their authority the unrelenting cold invaded through my clothes.

Brady was on the phone, but he hung up as soon as I entered the little dark apartment. As he came down the hall my once little boy towered over me. He saw himself as strong, but I saw how vulnerable he was. "Don't worry, Mom. He'll be all right," he said hopefully.

"Of course he will be, sweetie. You were a real trouper with the IV and all. I'm impressed that you reported it to the nurses in German."

"Well, I pointed a lot. It wasn't hard to see the problem. It turned out OK, didn't it?"

"Yes. Everything's OK," I said, and I hugged Ned's worried brother. "Ned is asleep and he'll be better in the morning. I'm the one with the problems, but that's nothing new! I'll work it out."

Brady laughed with relief. "No, that's nothing new," he teased and retired to his room.

E-mail was not enough. I waited long after Brady slept until I could catch Rick at home. My telephone call reached him at the end of a grueling day. He was exhausted and entangled in his work, which was much too far away for me to understand. All I could register was Ned and the situation in the Otto-Hoffen-Heim.

I blurted out the problem with the catheter and the accompanying complications. My news completely blindsided Ned's father. "But Pa died like that! He was in a hospital and he got an infection!" Rick cried. It was true, Rick's father did die of a postoperative infection, but I had not made the connection.

I rushed to comfort my husband. "Yes, darling. But Pa was a very sick and old man. He had had a really major operation. Ned is young and healthy, and the operation was on his left elbow. He has a fever, but he will be fine."

And so I found myself offering comfort where I felt none, reassuring where I felt no assurance, muddying the clarity of our communication when we both needed it most. By the end of the conversation the thousands of miles between Rick and me were all too real. We wanted to console each other but telephone conversations tend to be as linear as the wires that carry them; having set out on the wrong track it was impossible to start again. We hung up, miserably and mutually alone.

That night, all night, I lay sleepless in the Villa Walther. At the time of the first operation, Dr. Waldemeyer had declared the situation serious, but I had not agreed. But now as I lay in bed my little boy was miles away, infected, and either in pain or in a drugged sleep. I did not know who was taking care of him and questioned how capable they were of doing so. I wanted him with me so I could look after him, but the very infection that the hospital allowed to develop made me doubt that it would be responsible to move him now.

Outside I heard the sharp crack and crash of a tree limb, exploded and felled by the cold. The ghosts of the *Kurfürsten* galloped down the Koenigsallee, scattering the poor and the powerless as they pursued their pleasures. Wild animals huddled in the woods. I huddled awake in my bed and stared at the enormity of motherhood.

Ärtze (Doctors)

Thursday, January 25

Finally the morning came. Brady was focused on his test as he ate his breakfast. I bundled myself up for the trek through the Grunewald, and left him spoon in hand, with Newton's laws of motion open in front of him. I was too focused on my purpose to register the woods around me as I strode back to the hospital.

Genie met me in the cafeteria, dressed to the nines with a long black coat over all. "Germans respect power," she explained. We nibbled on breakfast and plotted strategy. We were both clear that the infection meant that Ned needed hospital care: it was equally clear, however, that that care had to be considerably more responsive than what he had received the day before. With Dr. Waldemeyer gone, though, it was hard to know to whom we should make this position known. We agreed, for the sake of propriety, to start at the level of the ward doctor, but we doubted that we would get much satisfaction there. After we had tried it we would go to Dr. Kawalek.

Promptly at eight-thirty we went together to *Zimmer Eins*. Ned lay small and pale in his bed, his breakfast untouched by his side, a new IV dripping at the base of his right thumb. His eyes were surrounded by dark circles, his lips were chapped, he had a fever. He was thirsty, he said, but he had nothing to drink. Nor could he have drunk it if he had, since his left arm was splinted, his right hooked to the IV.

Genie sprang into action. "First things first," she said and swooped off to get him some mineral water from the kitchen on the floor. As we went in to fetch it, a whey-faced successor to Big Nurz descended on us and ordered us out of the kitchen.

"The child is thirsty," Genie insisted, ignoring the command. "He needs water." She took a bottle from the crate and headed toward Ned.

"You may not do that!" the angry nurse shouted.

"Why not?" I asked, in case there was some kind of medical issue involved in giving Ned water.

"Parents are not allowed in the kitchen," she replied.

By that time we were out of the kitchen so I deemed her objection irrelevant. The tension, however, did not abate. Other nurses joined in to question our action.

"The child is thirsty," I explained in my short declarative German style. "He wants something to drink. He cannot do it alone. He is sick. He has a fever. He cannot get out of bed. He cannot hold the glass. He is helpless. He needs someone to help him."

"*Ja!*" a young nurse replied. "He is sick and in a hospital. We know what he needs."

I had come to the end of the line with my German. At just about this moment the doctor arrived. It was a different female doctor; not Dr. von Lennert, but one with bobbed hair. Genie went immediately on the offensive.

"*Ich heisse Eugenia Morgan,*" she said holding out her hand. "My name is Eugenia Morgan. And yours?"

The doctor was stunned and not pleased. "*Dr. Vierke,*" she said as she shook Genie's hand.

The conversation never warmed up from there. Genie asked for a clarification of what had happened the day before, why Ned had been neglected for so long. It turned out that Dr. Vierke had been the doctor in charge of the ward for the long morning of his pain and infection. She said she had asked that his catheter be removed at nine and it was not her fault that it was not. "*Normalerweise würde ein Arzt in einer Stunde heir sein.* Normally a doctor would have been here within the hour," she said. She and Genie went on leaving me in the dust of their German. I kept hearing the word *Normalerweise,* normally. I did not believe it. I had been told before about the turnaround time of the doctors on call and it was often not an hour. *Normalerweise.* I got angrier each time she said it.

The conversation moved to the present and Ned's current situation. Dr. Vierke moved to defend the nurses' care of Ned who, she declared, was quite capable of getting himself water if he was thirsty. Genie walked through the problems point by point: he was bed-bound by the IV, he could use neither arm. The issue moved to the bell—why had he not rung it? I pointed out that he could not use his arms to reach for a bell, but the observation proved superfluous when the nurse admitted he did not have one.

"Why not?" Dr. Vierke asked, truly boxed in this time.

"It is broken," the nurse confessed.

"He must have a bell!" Dr. Vierke commanded. She moved to the next bed.

Genie and I went outside. We were both furiously upset, but it was too cold to indulge ourselves for long; there was danger the tears would freeze on our cheeks. We took ourselves in hand and set off to find Dr. Kawalek. He was in surgery. Genie left her very impressive business card with crisp instructions to call as soon as he emerged. Then she had to go to work.

I went back to stand guard over Ned. I turned off the ubiquitous TV whenever his roommates left the room; when they were there I ran interference between him and the noisy, demanding six-year-old in the next bed. I read, either to him or, when he was too tired, to myself. When Petra came I paced the *Naturschutzgebiet*. Through it all the IV dripped its antibiotics into Ned's right arm. His fever subsided and he began to feel better.

I was supposed to be having lunch with Rudolf. I went so far as to catch the bus, but when I reached my stop I just crossed the street, called my apologies from a pay phone, and caught the bus returning. Ned was feeling better, but I was not at all secure in his position. I needed some kind of reassurance I had not yet received.

Ned was peacefully asleep. He did not need me at his side. So I went out to reconnoiter. It was lunchtime, so I was not allowed into the cafeteria to assuage my hunger. Dr. Kawalek was due to be out of surgery at one, but I had little hope he would talk to me immediately thereafter. In any case, I knew that all surgical times were infinitely negotiable. I paced the Otto-Hoffen-Heim, needing someone to talk to, having no idea who could fit the bill. Finally, in desperation, I decided to write a note to Dr. Heller. Fifteen minutes of his time would enable me to ask my questions of a doctor who was not enmeshed in the particulars of the case but who knew the hospital and its workings. I perched on the stairs of the main building and began to write him my request that he contact me on Station H.

As I was composing the missive, Frau Sonntag, a physical therapist who had occasionally filled in for Sigrid before the operation, came by and asked how Ned was doing. She was so warm and caring in her question that the last of my defenses crashed. I burst into tears. Frau Sonntag listened to my teary tale in broken German and instantly mobilized her forces to help. I needed an *Oberarzt,* and she bore me off to the one she had access to: the *Oberarzt* in charge of outpatient physical therapy.

Leaving me in the hall, Frau Sonntag went into her boss's office to explain the situation. Sigrid also went to talk to him between patients. I, on the other hand, was not invited in. The man would not speak a word to me because, with Ned on Station H, I was not under his purview. He did, however, make a number of phone calls, first to Station H and then to others of his colleagues. After I had waited for about fifteen minutes, Frau Sonntag assured me that the situation was well under control, that I should go back to Station H.

Comforted by the effort, though with no concrete results in hand, I went back to Ned's bedside. He had eaten what he wanted of his lunch so I picked at the edges to tide me over until the cafeteria reopened. He was cheery: with his roommates gone to some activity or another he had been able to turn off the irritating television. He snuggled against me as I read. We both began to feel better. Petra arrived to work his arm and I went down to read by the hot drinks machine.

I had not been there long when a nurse came down with the message that I was to go to the surgical admitting room. Dr. Kawalek's schedule had changed, and he was going to be in the operating room all day. Nonetheless he wanted to talk to me. She led me down the path and through the doors that had been closed on me in the past.

We entered a large, dim, dead-end corridor. Most of its left wall was a window through which I could see my hall's mirror image; that hall led into the operating theaters. When the nurse brought me in, a child was in the process of being moved from her rolling bed, through a robotically opened window, and onto a dolly on the other side. Before the window closed again, my sponsoring nurse told the orderly that I was there to speak with Dr. Kawalek. She left on my side of wall, he wheeled the child away on his. Alone, I hoped I would not be kept waiting too long in this surreal situation.

Dr. Kawalek did not keep me waiting, though. In minutes he appeared in green surgical scrubs. He opened a door next to the window, so that we were breathing the same air. He pulled his mask down so I could see he had a nose and a mouth. Mostly, though, I could see his eyes, which were gray-green and calm. "Hello, Mrs. Richards," he said in heavily accented English. "You want to talk with me about your son. You have problems on Station H?"

I was infinitely relieved. It was a strange environment, but I had gotten what I wanted; I was finally able to tell someone who had both power and perspective, what I saw as happening to Ned. I told Dr. Kawalek as succinctly as I could about what had happened the day before. He listened attentively and then began to explain about the hospital system for covering the wards. It was a story I had heard before. "Normally it is at most an hour before someone can come," he said.

"Normally, *Normalerweise*," in either language the word was like a red flag to my inner bull. "Normal it might be," I said, "but not for Ned. Not for Ned yesterday and not for him at other times as well."

"Other times?" he asked, and I told about the times we had waited hours to get the anesthetic syringe changed. "If you were his father, would you be comforted by the assurance that his experiences here were not normal? If you were me, would you leave matters to the staff of this hospital and go home to read a good book?"

"No, I wouldn't," Dr. Kawalek said gravely. "I would be doing just what you are doing."

"Would you leave him in this hospital?" I asked.

"Yes," he said. "He has an infection and needs to stay here at least until Monday. Then you can take him out, if you still want to." I accepted his position.

He went on: "I am here all day, and I cannot take care of Ned. I make sure someone does, however. Also I find a doctor who can talk to you and help you to deal with the hospital. I want to correct the bad impression we have made."

"Thank you," I said and we nodded to each other. I don't know the reality of the situation, but it seemed wrong to shake the hand of someone dressed as he was and he did not proffer one. He disappeared down the surgical corridor, and I retraced my steps—through the door, down the elevator, down the path, and into Station H. I slumped, exhausted but relieved, into a chair by the hot drinks machine.

Soon after that, Dr. Vierke bustled past carrying a large medical folder. I knew, without being told, that she was carrying Ned's records, if not to Dr. Kawalek, to someone he had appointed. About half an hour later she came back and I was proved right. She sat down next to me and asked about Ned's situation. She was a markedly different person than the one Genie had confronted five hours before.

Our conversation was in German. First, we went over the developments of the day before and tried to figure out what had gone wrong. Again we went through the party line about the response time of attending doctors, but Dr. Vierke admitted that it had not worked. I then questioned her about who had changed the syringe without responding to the problem that made the change irrelevant, if not pernicious. Here the conversation became more convoluted.

"*Wer hat die Spritze gewechselt?* Who changed the syringe?" I asked.

"VER*wechselt*," she corrected me.

VER*wechselt?* Ver- means wrong or strong. I just wanted to say: "Who changed the syringe?" Well, maybe the *ver* could be used to say "changed but shouldn't have been."

"*OK. Wer hat die Spritze verwechselt?*"

"*Weiss ich nicht.* I don't know," she responded. "*Ich frage.* I will ask."

I realized that I had really not asked the right question. I did not really care who had changed the syringe, but rather why someone with the authority to change it—a doctor—did not know that he or she was supposed to take out the catheter. I tried again to explain.

"*Es ist nicht wichtige* WER *die Spritze gewechselt hat. Was wichtig ist, ist* WARUM *man die Spritze gewechselt hat. Man hätte den Katheter abnehmen sollen. Statt dessen ist die Spritze gewechselt worden. Warum hat er nichts von dem Problem mit dem Katheter gewusst?*" ["It is not important WHO changed the syringe. What is important is WHY the syringe was changed. Someone should have known that the catheter should have been taken out. Instead the syringe was changed. Why didn't he respond to the problem with the catheter?"]

"VER*wechselt.*"

Damn this language and this woman.

"OK. VER*wechselt.*"

"*Ich frage.* I will ask."

We parted civilly and she went upstairs to conduct her investigations into Ned's treatment. I looked up *verwechseln* in my pocket dictionary and found that it meant "to mix up." Under no construction that I could make out was this the word I wanted to use when asking my questions. Ned's syringe had been changed, not mixed up. Since, in the event, Dr. Vierke never reported anything to me, I will never know what she investigated or what she found out.

Soon after my conversation with Dr. Vierke, Mrs. Harkin walked into *Zimmer Eins* full of the no-nonsense purpose that had carried her successfully through twenty years of fifth-grade teaching. Ned had used up the ten days projected by Dr. Waldemeyer for his stay. He had been absent long enough.

But even Mrs. Harkin was startled by the skinny, pale little boy in the bed with an IV in one arm and a huge splint on the other, who bore virtually no relation to the rambunctious youth who had trotted out of her classroom less than two weeks before. She stood at the end of Ned's bed, aghast.

"Ned, we miss you," she said simply. "We all miss you. We want you to get better as soon as you can. We want you to come back to us soon as you can."

Ned lay propped in his bed, awed by this visitation. "Yes, Mrs. Harkin," he said. "I am trying. I want to come back soon."

"You do just what the doctors tell you to do. They will make you well and then you can come back."

"Yes, Mrs. Harkin. I will," Ned said solemnly.

Waves of guilt washed over me. What had I allowed to happen to her pupil, my child? Was a left arm worth all of this? What was a left arm anyway? How was it to be weighed against a child's health? fifth-grade curriculum? a fifth-grade year? a sabbatical year?

I walked with Mrs. Harkin to the bus stop but found no answers in our conversation, which turned on my teaching Ned division so he would not fall hopelessly behind in mathematics. "Take care!" she said as she left.

"Thank you," I said. "I'll try."

It was Thursday night, usually dinner at the *Wissenschaftskolleg*. But this week had been special. Günther Grass had been at the *Kolleg* while I was tangling with Dr. von Lennert. Weeks later, when I was again noticing such things, a German fellow tried to comfort me for my loss. "His German was so convoluted even I had trouble following."

More immediately, Grass's Wednesday appearance meant that Thursday evening was free, and early in January, Helge had set up an evening at the symphony. She was clear that it was important that I keep things in perspective and continue with my life. "It is ten days from the operation. Ned will be home. He and Matteus can stay with Brady. We can go out," she firmly planned.

Left to my own devices, I had missed Günther Grass, but Helge was in charge of this evening and I did not have the strength to resist. Christopher had volunteered to stay with Ned so that I could feel secure during my night away. He arrived at five-thirty. I could see that the twins' father was as appalled as Mrs. Harkin had been by Ned's condition, but there was really nothing to say. He settled into the chair next to the sleeping Ned's bed and opened his book.

A man in *Zimmer Eins* was an occasion. The mothers watched in awe. The nurses did not ask him to move out of their way; in fact, one offered him a glass of water. Ned was in good hands. I left.

The Berlin Philharmonic Hall, the Philharmonie, is among the best concert halls in the world. It seats over a thousand, but so artfully that one has no sense of participating in a mass event. The audience is broken into sections that seem to float around the orchestra. The acoustics are excellent; even those in the cheap seats that go for less than twenty dollars can hear beautifully. Week after week the world's greatest performers pour their riches out for hundreds of Berliners. This evening I was with them and heard Mozart played by Murray Perahia.

I sat still next to Helge and tried to be carried away. I heard the notes but they refused to come together into melody and message. They jumbled incoherently around me.

> . . . this
> Is crumbled out again to his Atomies.

I recognized the snippet as another piece of the poem that had visited me the day before. I flipped mentally through all the poems I'd memorized for Grandmama, but I could neither complete nor place it. Nor could I put it aside. All entangled with the poem, Ned and his situation clambered for my attention and drowned out all music.

Friday, January 26

By eight-thirty the next morning, I had sent reassuring e-mail to Rick, roused and fed Brady, walked through the Grunewald, breakfasted with my paper, and was again at Ned's bedside. This morning it was Dr. von Lennert on rounds, accompanied by a quiet doctor I had seen once or twice before. Dr. von Lennert had long been convinced that my German was just fine and she always used it in our conversations. This morning she launched briskly into a long disquisition about Ned. I gathered that after visiting hours the night before, his bed had been the scene of a veritable mini-conference. Dr. Kawalek had come with Dr. Reisner, the *Oberarzt* in charge of anesthesiology, and Professor Mahler, the *Chefarzt*. This cast of characters was impressive indeed; in my wildest dreams I would never have expected Professor Mahler to visit Ned's bed. She said a great deal more that I did not understand, but I had spent enough time in the Otto-Hoffen-Heim to know that what I had heard was enough. As long as the "big boys" were on Ned's case he would be well taken care of.

Ned, for his part, was doing well. His fever was down, his medications seemed adequate to insure that he was not in real pain but were not so strong as to put him to sleep, and he was proud of the basket he was making in occupational therapy. Most of all there was Petra. Now that he was feeling better, Ned and she had begun to watch cartoons together. His favorite featured a baby chicken whose hat was the top of his eggshell. "*Calimero mit Sombrero*" was his name. "See, Mom! It's so cool! His name has three different languages in only three words. *Calimero* is Greek, *mit* is German, and *Sombrero* is Spanish."

❋ ❋ ❋

I hung around the edges of the action for a couple of hours but then left for lunch at the *Wissenschaftskolleg*. The expedition was basically an excuse that allowed me some freedom to let off steam. It was difficult for me to keep myself appropriately still in *Zimmer Eins*.

At lunch, I found it was equally difficult to match the ambience of the *Wissenschaftskolleg*. I tried not to overpower with my stories, to be quiet and listen to my colleague's conversation. But my experiences in the hospital had left me a coiled spring of pent-up anxieties, and after the meal I burst out of the *Kolleg* onto the frozen streets. Waiting for a bus was more than I could stand, so I walked several miles of the route until I intersected one at its stop.

In *Zimmer Eins*, Ned's eyes were regaining their twinkle, and he was ready to play cards. I held myself still by his bedside through a quiet afternoon of rummy, reading, and physical therapy.

At about four-thirty Beth arrived with the twins to cheer Ned up and lend me support. However, two 3-year-olds in the skinny space between ward beds was not a viable concept. Fortunately it was between doses of antibiotics, and with the catheter gone, this meant that Ned was free to get out of bed. So we all went down to the hot drinks machine where there was more space to play about. Just as we were settling down, a figure whose white legs beneath his parka revealed him as medical, came striding into view toward Station H. When he was still far away I recognized the blond curls and cheerful visage of Dr. Heller. He came in and asked whether this was a time that we could talk; Dr. Kawalek had designated him to be my medical liaison.

I don't know when I have been so glad to see anyone. I was absolutely desperate to talk to someone about our experience in the hospital. That Dr. Kawalek had selected Dr. Heller from a pool that could as easily have yielded either Dr. von Lennert or Dr. Vierke was a mark of his humane genius. I excused myself from the cheerful crowd of children while the young doctor found a key to Dr. Waldemeyer's office. We settled down on either side of the large desk.

I tried to be calm and to ask the kinds of medical questions a doctor is trained to answer. Although he had not been on the ground for most of it, Dr. Heller had been fully briefed about Ned's case. In the first five minutes of our conversation he spoke clearly to my questions about the catheter, the infection, the on-call system, the nurses' position in the hospital. I found myself quickly bored with the topics. I had been over the ground enough and Ned's improving condition meant that it was no longer compelling.

After I'd touched all of the required bases, neither of us was satisfied. "You still seem upset," he said. "I can show you on Ned's chart how his fever is going down. Would that help?" He smiled hopefully beneath his cherubic curls.

"Oh, Dr. Heller," I blurted. "You have no idea what it is like to be a mother on Station H! It's as if . . ."

The door to the office opened. Dr. Vierke came in and began to look for something in the file cabinets. Dr. Heller expected me to continue, but I had closed like a clam. He looked up, registered the problem, and grinned conspiratorially. "So," he said, "a fever like Ned's indicates a problem but it is not terribly serious. It goes down with the antibiotics. In a week I am sure he is completely healthy again."

"Yes," Dr. Vierke offered, found folder under her arm. "It is not a problem."

"Good," I said carefully.

"You were going to tell me about being a mother on Station H," Dr Heller prompted me as his colleague closed the door behind her. Her interruption had given me a moment to reflect.

"It's OK," I said. "You are not a psychologist. It's not your job to worry about how I feel."

"Dr. Kawalek told me to talk to you," the young man replied. "And I am studying to be a child's doctor. It is good for me to know how it feels to be a mother on Station H."

That was enough. My confused frustrations poured out of me, on and on. "Ned was really sick, but no one cared! The nurses were hopeless! They stood around and made phone calls but no one did anything about it! *'Frau Richards, ein Arzt kommt,* a doctor comes.' Ya, right! A doctor is coming. We have already called. So I'm supposed to shut up. But no one did anything. Not for ten minutes, not for twenty minutes, not for hours! For hours and hours and hours! The whole hospital just stood around until I blew my stack! Then they act as if I am weird.

"And everyone is so rude! They don't listen! They don't explain anything! They yell at me when I ask questions! They don't do what they say they are going to do! I feel so helpless. I feel so ignored. I feel as if I don't exist. I know my German is poor, but if people slow down I can usually follow. If people talk to me I *always* listen. Ned has been really sick. But they don't explain. They don't talk to me at all. No one will even tell me his name!"

I spoke quickly and passionately, and I doubt that Dr. Heller understood every word. But it was such a wonderful relief just to let fly that I did not care particularly. "They come into the room and they don't even look at me. They don't look at Ned either. They just manhandle him and stick him with needles and then they leave. They don't ask what is up. They don't explain what they are doing. They won't even tell me their names!"

When the flood of words ceased there was a brief silence. However much he had understood, Dr. Heller could not deal with the whole. He murmured sympathetically and found a focus. "We Germans do not always tell our names. Maybe it is because we are afraid to be responsible. Let me try to help." He drew a chart with Professor Mahler in charge of Orthopedics, Dr. Reisner in charge of Anesthesiology. Below was a second tier of *Oberärzte,* including Drs. Waldemeyer and Kawalek; he then moved to a third tier, of advanced residents, that included himself as well as Drs. Vierke and von Lennert. As he talked and diagrammed, he slowly realized that he was not really addressing the issue. I knew the names and the positions he was telling me. It was the people who corresponded to them that I did not know.

Dr. Heller changed his tack. "Dr. Reisner? He was with Professor Mahler when he visited Ned last night."

"But I wasn't," I pointed out.

"Why not?" he asked, a bit surprised by my cavalier approach to the *Chefarzt*.

"Nobody told me they were coming," I replied.

We went on. "Well, you know Professor Mahler."

"No, I don't," I contradicted.

"Yes, you do. He is the man who canceled Ned's operation before Christmas." I was coming across as mentally deficient.

"But Dr. Waldemeyer relayed that message to me on the telephone. Professor Mahler never talked to me. I don't know who Professor Mahler *is*."

My ignorance was total, and Dr. Heller was stymied. Without points of reference at the top of the hierarchy he could not locate the people with whom I had been dealing. We tried to approach the problem from the other direction. I felt like the host of some kind of quiz show as I posed my question.

"Who is the anesthesiologist who is always so cheerful? He wears glasses, does not have long hair, and his English is not particularly good."

Dr. Heller grinned as he admitted he had no idea. "I don't know what kind of English the anesthesiologists speak," he pointed out.

"Who is the quiet man with salt-and-pepper hair—that means mixed white and black hair—who was with Dr. von Lennert on rounds this morning?" I tried.

This time he hit the jackpot. "That was Dr. Kawalek," he said. "But you *have* met him!"

"Yes, I have, but only in surgical scrubs! I saw only his eyes then; he had a green hat on. It was his hair that I saw this morning." I sat a moment embarrassed. That morning I had been trying so hard to follow Dr. von Lennert's German I had ignored Dr. Kawalek entirely. "I can't do anything in the hospital if I never know who I'm talking to. It's not just that I don't know who is responsible for any given situation. I can't even thank people who have been helpful!"

"Our system is hard for you to understand," Dr. Heller observed, and he promised to take up the issue of names with the orthopedic group. I understood enough to know that it was simply ridiculous to think that in this rigid hierarchy a doctor at his level could have any effect on the practice of the medical staff. Still, I was grateful that he said he would try, and his listening had done me a great deal of good.

As we got up to go I asked the young doctor. "Will you please give me your telephone number?" He looked at me, aghast. "I promise I will not use it unless there is something really desperate going on," I said. "But the nurses say Dr. Waldemeyer will not be back until Monday and they are so completely helpless if there is a problem. I just need to know that there is somewhere I could call if I had to."

Dr. Heller slowly wrote a number on a slip of paper, and handed it to me. Without peeking, I stuck it between the pages of the little yellow notebook. "Thank you," I said. "I promise I won't use it."

His pause had given him a moment to reflect and he grinned his understanding. "You may use it if you need to," he said.

Our conversation had taken almost an hour, which was a long time for Beth and the children. As soon as it was over, we bundled up the jabbering twins, and she herded them into the freezing night. Ned and I returned to his room upstairs. I was calm in a way I hadn't been for weeks. Finally, I had penetrated the slippery façade of the Otto-Hoffen-Heim and actually made contact with some real people. When one of them failed me I could turn to another. I could find rest in Dr. Kawalek's responsive calm, sympathy in Dr. Heller's youthful openness, adventure in Dr. Waldemeyer's sparkling dash. I had located the coordinates of a comfortable place for me in the Otto-Hoffen-Heim. Ned and I settled cozily on his bed with a book.

The day's action was not over, though; we had not read more than a page when Dr. Waldemeyer came in. For the first time in months I was not elated to see him. My experiences with Drs. Kawalek and Heller had left me satisfied and I felt no particular need to talk further. Still I roused myself to speak to him alone. I had certainly stirred the pot in his absence; it seemed only fair to warn him.

"When you were gone I had a fit," I confessed in the hall outside of the room.

My choice of words, with its resonance to seizures, was unfortunate and the man was startled. "You did what?" he asked.

"I got upset," I explained. "You were not here and I was worried about Ned. I talked to a lot of people about it."

"You talked to a lot of people?" he queried, still somewhat perplexed. "Who?"

I gave him the basic outlines of my action during the time he was away. He listened carefully. "That was right. Ned is not his patient," he judged when I said that the doctor in physical therapy had not spoken to me. "Yes, that was right, I put him in charge," he noted when I said I had spoken to Dr. Kawalek. "*Professor* Mahler," he corrected me when I said Dr. Mahler had been to see Ned. "Yes, Dr. Kawalek told him to," he commented when I told him of speaking with Dr. Heller. The returning *Oberarzt* kept my two-day saga a totally institutional one. He had left me to the care of a system; at the end of my exposition he seemed satisfied that I had not violated any of the basic rules. "That was all right," he concluded. "But now I am back. You do not need the others anymore. I take care of Ned."

Dr. Waldemeyer was as good as his word. In the rest of Ned's time at the Otto-Hoffen-Heim I spoke with Dr. Heller only in passing. I never again spoke to Dr. Kawalek, although that night I did write him a note.

27.01.96

Dear Dr. Kawalek,

I want to thank you for taking such good care of a mother in distress. In the first place, that involved taking care of her son. I can see that the medical staff is on top of Ned's condition and that he is getting better. In this case, it also involved finding someone within the hospital I could talk to. Dr. Heller has been very helpful.

Even as I write I want to apologize for being so late and indirect with these thanks. One of the issues I discussed with Dr. Heller is that I do not know the names of the medical staff in the Otto-Hoffen-Heim. This means that often I do not know to whom I am speaking. In particular, I did not know that the quiet, attentive man with Dr. von Lennert this morning was the same person I had seen in surgical scrubs the day before. Had I known that it was you I would have thanked you in person; as it is, I thank you now.

Sincerely yours,
Joan L. Richards

Camp Oh-Ha-Ha

At eight-thirty the next day, after I'd delivered Dr. Kawalek's note to the hospital post office, I went to Station H. I expected all to be calm. Instead I found Ned surrounded by an episode of doctors who were trying to find a place in his right arm to insert yet another IV. There were two infusions on their stands waiting to be dripped into him but the shunt in the base of his thumb had given out during the night. Even Dr. von Lennert murmured sympathetic assent when I pointed out that Ned was small, young, and sick, his right arm a mass of bruises from blood tests and IVs.

"Can't you give him the antibiotics orally?" I asked.

"That would be a lot of pills," the unnamed man in charge replied.

"He can take pills," I assured him.

The probing doctors were skeptical and kept searching for a promising vein. When two additional tries failed, however, even they gave up. The infusions were wheeled away and Ned began taking pills at a terrific rate. At last he was free of his IVs. For the first time in almost two weeks he could walk around at will.

The same morning Ned and Hans, the whiny child in the next bed, reached the end of their collective rope. The immediate issue concerned the television. The crowd of vein-searching doctors had interrupted a concerted campaign that Ned contribute his fair share to television viewing by buying a telephone chip. As soon as they left, Hans began again to demand twenty marks. Ned, for whom it was a toss-up which had been more irritating—the insistent voice that was hammering at him even as it had throughout his fever, or the equally persistent sound of the television—refused. By the time I arrived, their conflict was explosive. My attempt to defuse it by buying the television chip failed when the machine swallowed my money. In desperation I explained the situation to the nurses and left them to deal with it. I had to go shopping.

By the time I got back at around noon Ned had been moved to *Zimmer Zwei*, and the ward was calm. Ned's new roommates were Herbert and Erik, both of whom were about his age. They were often joined by Karim, a sweet Egyptian boy from *Zimmer Eins*. I came to see the foursome as the center of Camp Oh-Ha-Ha, a name I generated from the German pronunciation of the initials of Otto-Hoffen-Heim. Their counselors were the physical and occupational therapists who worked closely with all of them. Also important was Dieter, a nurse in training. He was a comfort to Ned because he spoke English. When not otherwise engaged, Dieter actually spent time in *Zimmer Zwei* doing things like simultaneously playing two games of chess in two different languages. He was a welcome male presence for the boys on the ward.

When Brady arrived that Saturday afternoon I left my children to negotiate the new social world together. I was glad that Ned was mobile and in a room that smacked as much of a winter camp as a hospital. Still, it had been eleven days since his operation. According to Dr. Waldemeyer's original projection, Ned should have been at home working his basically mobile arm in an outpatient physical therapy regime. Instead he was, as far as I could tell, the sickest child in Camp Oh-Ha-Ha. I was tired, spent, and grateful for the anonymity of the hot drinks machine.

It was quiet there; no one else was around and the trees around the Otto-Hoffen-Heim glistened in the frigid sunlight. I was just settling down when Dr. von Lennert appeared from upstairs, accompanied by another unknown doctor. To my surprise, they did not proceed outside but came to me. I stood up and Dr. von Lennert introduced me to Professor Mahler. We shook hands and Professor Mahler began to speak in beautifully intoned German. He was used to public speaking, but I did not hear what he said after the first few sentences. *"Sie können Ned noch nicht mit nach Hause nehmen. Er muss noch zwei oder drei Wochen bei uns bleiben. Sein Ellbogen ist schwer verletzt. Er wird nie wieder normal werden. Ihr Sohn wird behindert bleiben, aber wir wollen dass er die grössest mögliche Bewegungsfreiheit hat. Dazu ist es unbedingt erforderlich dass er länger hier bleibt."* ["You cannot take Ned home yet. He must stay here for two or three more weeks. His elbow has been very badly hurt. It will never be normal again. Your son will remain handicapped, but we want him to have the greatest possible mobility. That is why it is imperative that he stay here longer."]

My thoughts flew to my beautiful, joyous little boy, my *federnd*, irrepressible Ned. I saw him running, swimming, playing—wild and free. Now he was going to be *behindert*, handicapped, struggling all his life with the most basic tasks, unable even to button a shirt. I was expected to respond. I made no attempt to do so in German; to do so in English required all of my inner resources. Picking up on the most neutral thing I had understood, I said "two or three more weeks here? That is impossible. He has already been here for two. He has to come home." Professor Mahler's English was not as sonorous as his German but he could certainly carry on a conversation in it. He had said his piece in his language, we could discuss trivialities in mine. We talked back and forth about his projections for Ned's stay: about my circumstances in Germany, my fellowship, Brady, our living situation.

After a decent interval of discourse, Professor Mahler and Dr. von Lennert walked out into the frozen day. He said something to her, and she looked up at him, laughing, as they traversed the path toward the main hospital building. The scene etched itself indelibly in my mind. It was not just the contrast of her laughter with the pain of the conversation we had just had, though that was real. It was her whole orientation, slightly turned in the *Chefarzt's* direction as they strode along, looking up into his face. He was the focus of her attention—both the model to which she aspired and the key to her success. Ned and his arm were at best a distraction.

Throughout the weekend Dr. Waldemeyer was very conscientious; although he was technically still off duty he passed through to check on Ned every day. I did not know what the implications were for him of Ned's situation; certainly all the fuss I had made could not have made life among his colleagues easier. Professor Mahler's *"behindert"* was devastating for me to hear, but it might equally have been aimed at an upstart underling who went ahead with a risky operation when he should have held back. I really wanted to talk to Dr. Waldemeyer about the whole situation in which we found ourselves. I wanted to talk to him about the implications of what had happened—of the infection, of the time lost to Ned's pain, of his stiffening arm. I wanted to understand the past so we could work together into the future.

Dr. Waldemeyer's carefully controlled five-minute appearances did little to help me in my struggle to understand. He smiled carefully at me in my seat by Ned's side and posted himself at the end of the bed. "Ned, you must move the arm. It is very important. You must move it and move it and move it and move it. I cannot do it for you. Your mother cannot do it for you. It is your arm and you must move it."

Ned sat politely still, his splinted arm at his side. "OK," he said.

The doctor again smiled and left.

On Sunday I followed him out of the room.

"Yes?" Dr. Waldemeyer was never rude to me but he did have a freeze mode for conversations he did not want to have, and he was in it now. "Did you want to speak with me?"

I groped for an opening. What could I ask? How could I ask how to understand?

"I'm confused," I tried. "What is happening?"

"What is happening?" He echoed my question coolly.

"Yes, what is happening? What is going on with Ned's arm? Sitting here day after day is driving me absolutely crazy. Is the elbow getting better?"

"There is nothing new about this. I told you he would have to move his elbow. The operation will not work unless he does."

"But how long will we have to be here?"

"Until it is better! He has to move it and move it and move it. We see when it is better."

"But it has already been almost two weeks!"

"So? It is hard for me too. It is hard for my family because I come every day here to see Ned. I did not tell you it would be easy and I do not know how long it is."

I was effectively silenced. When he saw that I was not going to *schimpfen* with him about the hospital or the infection, he warmed slightly: "It is easier for me to say it than for you to do it."

"Yes, it is. But I see your point and you should go."

He smiled happily: "We skate on the Wannsee!"

Engulfed with a wave of longing, I grasped for my manners. "What fun!" I said. "Have a good time."

"Yes!" Eyes sparkling with anticipation, the doctor wrapped his scarf around his neck. His frizzy curls bounced as he strode away.

Petra had taken the weekend shift so she could keep working with Ned's arm. Ned called her his "physical terrorist," the perfect term for a German physical therapist for whom the sound *th* was unpronounceable.

"Hey, Ned! We get 130 degrees today. Yes?"

"Y-Y-Yes!" he said, with just the right teen-aged inflection.

"Yes!" she copied and they got down to it.

But they did not get 130 degrees. Petra sat by Ned's side for hours, laughing at his jokes, playing with his German, teaching him physiology, and moving his arm. But by the end of the weekend, he could no longer put his hand in his jeans pocket nor could he comfortably touch his chin.

✿ ✿ ✿

At home that evening, Brady was on the phone, and I went, restless, to the office where I hadn't worked in weeks. I had come to Germany with such high hopes, so determined to put Ned's problems in perspective and keep my career on track. I had overridden Ned's homesickness, Brady's reluctance, and Rick's immobility with my clear-sighted purpose. Ned had trusted me, Brady had trusted me, Rick had trusted me. They had all changed their lives to fit my vision. I had been so sure.

Others had trusted me as well. All of those who had recommended me for the fellowship, and those who had given it to me. They had believed that I would do as I said. They had given me a chance.

I had tried so very hard. I had tried to be patient. I had tried to be reasonable. I had tried to be flexible. I had tried everything I could think of to make this year work, to keep writing, and to take care of Ned. But I was being defeated. Ned's arm did not work and my book was not being written. People tried to help, but it was not enough. I was alone, isolated, blocked everywhere I turned. The empty building was dark and silent around me.

The poem came to me. I realized that it was by John Donne. His distress in 1611 was over the replacement of the Aristotelian, earth-centered cosmos by the Copernican, Sun-centered one. A larger selection has long been standard fare in introductory history of science courses. I reached to the book on my shelf and looked it up:

> [The] new Philosophy calls all in doubt,
> The Element of fire is quite put out;
> The Sun is lost, and th'earth, and no man's wit
> Can well direct him where to look for it.
> And freely men confess that this world's spent,
> When in the Planets, and the Firmament
> They seek so many new; then see that this
> Is crumbled out again to his Atomies.
> 'Tis all in pieces, all coherence gone;
> All just supply and all Relation:
> Prince, Subject, Father, Son, are things forgot,
> For every man alone thinks he hath got
> To be a Phoenix. . . .

I comforted myself by thinking about Donne, about me. He was struggling to make sense of a world whose shape and character were being transformed by radical new ideas. Not only were new theories hurling the earth out of its place in the universe, they were crumbling its previously coherent substance into atomic discontinuities. Donne didn't know even how to begin to think in such a disordered universe.

I felt similarly lost. With each passing day in the Otto-Hoffen-Heim my understanding was coming apart at the seams. In a sense I was mourning the breakup of the world whose beginning Donne could not see. He did not realize how coherent the post-Copernican world could become; how comfortable for Newton and my Victorians, for Grand-mama, and, vicariously, for me. My experience was making me a traitor to their world where the public and private were sharply defined and not to be mixed. I had lost their clear understanding of the real and the unreal, of the certain and the uncertain, of truth and falsity.

Ever since Ned had his first seizure I had tried to adhere to the order of their vision; to stay calm and manage my life with Ned according to the rational, controlled principles they espoused. I was not going to stop now. I knew of no other way to proceed. But behind my proceeding I was lost. I was alone in a strange world that I did not understand. The manners of my Victorians were in place, but their effective confidence had deserted me entirely. I gazed through tears at the desk where I was supposed to work. I looked around the tiny office where only a few months ago I had planned to do so much. Now it was just an empty space, an unfulfilled hope. There was nothing I could do there. But Donne ended his poem with a phoenix, and phoenixes rise from their ashes. I shared neither his world nor his problems, but he did offer hope.

Whatever was to raise me was not going to appear at my desk this evening; I could not even pretend to work in the midst of all this. I washed my face in the bathroom at the end of the quiet, dark corridor. Then I walked back to the apartment and ruffled Brady's ever-longer hair as he lay reading a history book on the couch.

Schiene (Splints)

Early on Monday morning, Dr. Waldemeyer tried to move Ned's arm. I had initiated this experiment because I thought it was important for the doctor to get the feel of Ned's motion. But, in the event, mine was perhaps not a good idea. It was very hard for the surgeon to slow himself down enough to take on the problem. He grasped the little limb with such force that Ned's protesting yelps were as often directed at the surgeon's grip as at his elbow. *Locker lassen!* [Relax!] was an instruction both man and boy needed when they tried to work together.

After the struggle, in which Dr. Waldemeyer sadly noted how very restricted Ned's motion had become, he ordered a new bending splint. This was a move in an arena that had been static ever since the Wednesday after the operation when the cheery anesthesiologist had numbed Ned's arm in the surgeon's absence. Since then some tacit agreement seemed to have ruled the extending splint out of reach. Ned always wore the bending one between physical therapy sessions and at night. This now-graying friend held Ned's arm crooked comfortably at about 100 degrees, just slightly more than a right angle. The new one was to hold his arm bent to 125 degrees, which was considerably farther.

A blond nurse brought this instruction to Ned's bedside after Dr. Waldemeyer had left. I could see the logic behind it. If Ned were bent to his utmost all the time between physical therapy sessions, his flexion simply could not slip any further. Dr. Waldemeyer wanted to preserve his flexion at all costs. We went together to the *Gipsraum* and did our best to help Ned bend his arm to the doctor's specifications. "*Armes Kind,* poor child" the woman in the Gipsraum commented, as, after half an hour of struggle, we bore the punishingly tight bending splint back to the ward.

The nurse laid the new splint on the lockers to dry. Petra eyed it warily when she came for physical therapy sessions, but she made no comment. She was working on another scheme; she was out to get Ned a Dynasplint.

The advertising pictures Petra showed us were of a contraption, consisting of two hinged steel rods that could be strapped with faux leather sleeves to a child's upper and lower arms. The vital issue was the hinge at his elbow, which was springed and could be adjusted to apply more or less pressure to straighten the elbow. A Dynasplint is an expensive gadget; it cost on the order of 2,800 marks [about $2,100], but Petra and the physical therapists ascertained that Ned's insurance would pay for it. They ignored Dr. Waldemeyer's bending splint on the lockers and pressed their case for an extending Dynasplint with the hospital administration.

The Dynasplint arrived on Tuesday, and all the physical therapists stood around admiringly as Petra strapped it on and adjusted the spring with its special screwdriver. It was fun for Ned to experiment with a more mobile arm that was held extended but could be bent at will. He cheerily wore it for the first hour after each of his sessions with Petra; beyond that it made his arm ache and he traded it for his old favorite. Dr. Waldemeyer's bending splint lay untouched on the top of the lockers. "It's not dry yet!" Ned told me cheerily when I asked him about it.

But at about seven o'clock that evening, long after all physical therapists and doctors had left the scene, the blond nurse came to organize *Zimmer Zwei* for the night. In the midst of the usual dispensing of medications and instructions about pajamas and tooth brushings, she said briskly to Ned: "Tonight you must wear the new bending splint to sleep." She removed the familiar one from Ned's arm and brought down the one that had lain peacefully on the locker during the previous thirty-two hours.

Ned tried, but his arm did not bend far enough to fit into the tight angle. "I can't put it on," he said.

"You must exercise," she said firmly. "Dr. Waldemeyer says you must wear this splint in the night."

Ned jerked his arm up and down a couple of times "to warm it up." But it still came nowhere near to fitting into the bending splint. "Well," the nurse said firmly. "Dr. Waldemeyer says you must wear it. You must move your arm, Ned. I come back in fifteen minutes to put it on."

I was heartsick to see how difficult it was for Ned to bend his arm enough to put on the bending splint; it made it absolutely clear that he had lost ground even since the day before. But this was a situation in which I could help. I had seen enough physical therapy to have a sense of what was required to move Ned's arm. "OK, Ned! We can do it!" I said heartily, and settled myself at his side. "You show me what Petra does and we'll get you all set!"

Ned tried to cooperate by walking me through the basic procedure of bending and massage, but when the nurse returned about fifteen minutes later I had still not succeeded in putting his arm into the splint. As I bent the elbow on one side of the bed she tried to help Ned relax on the other. "*Atmen,* Ned! Breath!" she said gently, breathing deeply herself. "*Locker Lassen!* Relax!" I held Ned's arm while she forced the bending splint over his elbow. We secured it with the ace bandage.

"Will you read to me, Mom?" Ned asked pleadingly. It was an hour past the end of visiting hours, Herbert and Erik had long since settled into their television show, but the nurse indicated I could stay. Ned lay curled around his splinted arm and I read softly into his ear.

"Good night, sweetie," I said at the end of the chapter.

"Do you have to go, Mom?"

"Yes, it's late. I have to have dinner with Brady. Will you be all right?"

"Yes, I'll just go to sleep."

"Good night," I said again, but it did not ring true.

The next morning I arrived to a very interested and alert crew in *Zimmer Zwei.* Karim was there, Petra was there, a couple of nurses were there, and as I walked in I had the sense they had been lying in wait for me. Karim broke the silence.

"Ned say you are professor. *Frau Professor Doktor!* Is that right?"

"Yes," I told the listening crowd. "*Ja, ich bin Professorin.* I am a professor." It was not a time to explain the intricacies of the somewhat different American system in which I am a professor; that my position as an associate professor was closer to Dr. Waldemeyer as *privat dozent* than to the venerable Professor Mahler.

Ned beamed from his bed. "*So.* I told you," he said proudly in his best schoolboy German.

"*Stimmt!* It's true!" said the awed Karim. Herbert and Erik regarded Ned with somewhat confused respect.

I laughed inwardly as I sat down in my accustomed seat next to his bed. Ned really was getting better! Half an hour of showing off his ability to dive for submerged rings in *Hydrotherapie* might further contribute to his social standing. I helped him into my big-sleeved jacket, and put on his hat. He danced his circles around the others who variously limped and crutched down the hall.

Alone for the next half hour I found myself confronting Karim's surprise. I could see why the boys in Camp Oh-Ha-Ha had trouble with my status. There could not be a greater disparity in behavior than that between the crisp and hurried *Ärzte,* and *die Mutter von Ned,* Ned's mother, who sat through day after day on Station H. Their amazement illuminated with shocking clarity the situation I had been drawn into.

As I sat and waited for Ned to come back from *Hydrotherapie* I saw that my place was among the world of women and children on Station H. Frau Professor Doktor Richards lived in a different world where time could be measured and controlled. For the nonce she would just have to wait. I was going to have to do my thinking in and about the Otto-Hoffen-Heim and all that was happening there.

Ned returned. We read a bit. Petra came. I left to forage for lunch.

That night Ned and I again faced the bending splint. This time the blond nurse gave him an additional Tylenol an hour in advance. I then struggled for at least that long to squeeze his arm into the crooked plaster. As I triumphantly affixed it with its Ace bandage my poor child was in serious pain. *We'll just hold it here a minute. It will stop hurting if we just hold it.* I determinedly waited for Sigrid's promise to take effect, for the pain to subside as the arm lay still, but it did not. After ten minutes Ned was still curled around the arm, plucking obsessively at his protruding fingers.

"Please, Mom! Can't you take it off? It hurts! I am bent all the way in! Isn't that enough?"

"Yes. It is enough!" I unwrapped the bending splint and released Ned's arm. I had had enough of torturing Ned for the surgeon's ideas of what was required. He had no idea of how much it hurt.

On Friday Dr. Waldemeyer began to make plans to be out of town for his long-awaited conference. Ned was to be left under the care of Dr. Lützen, the advanced resident who routinely ran Station H. Before Dr. Waldemeyer disappeared, the three of us spent fifteen minutes going over the basic plan for the following week. I emerged comfortable that I knew who was in charge of Ned and clear about what was to happen: "We begin to taper the morphine so maybe Ned goes home on the weekend."

On Saturday Dr. Waldemeyer was gone, and Rick appeared, luggage bursting with English-language books and batteries. It was a great relief to have him there; I was ready for some help on Station H. But Rick was very poorly placed to help in the Otto-Hoffen-Heim. He had watched through the operation, suffered through the infection, and rejoiced when Ned's health returned. But the two of us had never really recovered from the wrong turn of the telephone call about Ned's fever.

Once I had taken the role of strong, reassuring comforter, it had been just too hard to backtrack. It had simply been easier to mask the ongoing drama and uncertainties in my e-mail.

For his part, Rick had been comfortable with the protection my approach afforded. He lived elsewhere and there was only so much of the German medical experience he could engage. He knew the measure of operation, fever, and movement, but was not in a position to deal with much more than that. So when he arrived in Berlin on a frigid Saturday in February, Rick was totally unprepared to find his family swallowed up by Ned's left elbow.

Even had it not been a woman's world, without German and the weeks of familiarity I had acquired, Rick would have found Ned's hospital ward a difficult place to be. But I was ready for some freedom, and all too happy to leave him there for days, playing cards with Ned and dealing with the nurses.

"Why don't you go to the hospital and I'll spend some time in my office."

"I came to be with *you,* Joan, to have some time with the family."

"I know. But I don't know what to *do* about it, Rick. There's no room for the two of us there, and we can't just leave him alone all the time."

"He's got to come home! This is ridiculous!"

But I couldn't even begin to bring Ned home. Dr. Waldemeyer was in Munich; neither Dr. Lützen nor I was in any position to change the agreement that the three of us had forged before Rick arrived. So he, Brady, and I went to the hospital to play hearts with Ned by the hot drinks machine.

After a couple of days negotiating jet lag and smoldering frustrations Rick and I began to recognize our plight as shared. This removed some of the tension, but it did not alleviate the harsh reality of our lives. We moved ceaselessly in the dark and frozen city, alone or together, on foot or on bus or impatiently waiting, seemingly always somewhere on the route between the Villa Walther and the Otto-Hoffen-Heim. Brady's vacationing life with his friends intersected ours sporadically— on buses, by Ned's bed, sometimes for dinner and an evening—but it could hardly be called family life. Rick was hurt, lost, and dislocated to the extreme.

Medically, the first part of the week proceeded according to plan; if anything the morphine taper went better than had been expected. Between Monday and Wednesday Ned gained ten degrees in both directions. He could touch his neck. Several finger tips fit into his jeans pocket. Things were improving dramatically!

Thursday was more problematic, however. Ned reported difficult physical therapy sessions without particularly good motion. I figured it was par for the course, one had to mix the bad with the good, and I let it go at that.

Thursday evening Rick and I had dinner at the *Wissenschaftskolleg*, my first Thursday night dinner in weeks. We left Ned's bedside early to enjoy every minute of it. Frau Breunig greeted Rick as we came in and he practiced his German with her while I sorted through my mail. It was good to enter an adult world with my husband at my side.

Then we went down for dinner. It was not children's night but Brady was happy to while away the evening on my office computer. Rick and I sat with the Wests and the McAllisters, all of us content to abandon the pretence of speaking any language but English.

As the meal progressed, Christopher and Rick plunged happily into conversation about public accountability in funding for education. I listened with half an ear, intrigued by the ways their analyses of accounting systems had been translated from historians looking at the social implications of scientific and technological ones. With another half ear I listened to Jane and Bill telling Beth about a trip they were going to take through Africa in pursuit of some of Jane's social interests. Just after we were married Rick and I actually ran an orphanage in Ethiopia for two years, and I was interested in the new world they were describing. With yet another half ear I listened to myself calming down—Ned was not an issue, I was still a viable member of this community, I could find ways to do my work.

As the meal was drawing to a close and I was reaching the point where I might even speak, Brady appeared, threading his long body among the various tables to my chair.

"Ned is on the phone, Mom. He wants to speak to you."

Damn!

"What does he want, Brady? Can't you talk to him?"

"Mom, he's really upset. I don't know what the problem is, but I think you'd better talk to him."

Damn, damn, damn, damn, DAMN!

I excused myself from the table, and went to the phone in my office.

"Hello," I said crisply.

"Mom! Mom!" Ned cried. "You've got to come! You've got to come right now. You have to help me, Mom!"

My mood changed in an instant, and I worked to calm Ned down. After a few minutes I began to piece the situation together. He was involved in a fight with Dieter; the hero of the ward was angry at him.

Dieter's problem was with whether Ned was moving his arm between physical therapy sessions. This had long been an area of slippage between the official line and actual practice. The doctors' scenario was that Ned would move his arm constantly as he sat in bed, but in his first postoperative week Ned had taken a firm stand that four or five sessions of physical therapy daily was enough pain and he was not going to augment it by moving his arm between Petra's visits. No one had confronted him about this and I often heard him reject supplemental pain medication on the grounds that since his arm was securely splinted at the moment it was not hurting him.

On this Thursday, however, Dieter was concerned about Ned's slipping angles. He had decided to enforce the movement regime and refused to bend to Ned's resistance. By the time Ned called me the young nurse had raised the ante. He had given Ned the task of exercising his arm to the point that it could be put into the bending splint for the night. Ned was in a panic.

I could understand the young nurse's position; he wanted Ned's arm to move more than it did and was backed by doctor's orders. I could also see Ned's position: I had watched him pluck desperately, obsessively, at the fingers protruding from the splint in a vain attempt to assuage his pain. I tried to calm Ned down and define a middle ground between the determined young man and my son.

"Why don't you bend it so that it *could* go into the splint," I suggested. "Just do it once to 120 degrees and that will take care of it."

"But Mom, he won't let me," Ned wailed. "He says I must wear it all night."

I got Dieter on the phone. He was completely clear about his position, and his determination was amply fueled by what he saw as Ned's laziness about moving his arm during the day.

"I do not want you to put Ned into that splint for the night," I insisted. "We can talk over the policy with the doctors in the morning, but for the moment I take responsibility for this decision. I have told Ned that he should work his arm very hard and do his best to get it into the cast. For the night he will wear the other splint, though."

The young man accepted my decision and gave the phone back to Ned. I told Ned what Dieter and I had agreed. He acquiesced, though unhappily, and asked that I not hang up. Then he put the phone down so Dieter could bend his arm.

I did not know how far he was from fitting in or I would never have given the young man permission to have his way with Ned's arm. Through the receiver I listened helplessly as the irritated nurse forced it into position.

"Is that all you can do? That is just 110 degrees!"

Ned cried out. "Stop! Stop! It hurts!"

"That is only 113 degrees," Dieter insisted.

One hundred fifteen degrees, 118 degrees, with each increment Ned's pain and resistance increased: Dieter stubbornly went on. "There! 120 degrees!" he crowed exultantly. Ned wept as Dieter's footsteps faded in the background.

How can you tell a child you are sorry on the telephone? I tried and then went, defeated, back to the table.

"What was that, Joan?" Jane asked, all clear, sharp, and in control.

"Oh, nothing. Ned was just a bit lonely." The real situation was simply too confusing to go into. After about five more polite minutes Rick, Brady, and I went back to the Villa Walther.

Erwachsene (Adults, Grown-Ups)

It was time to take Ned out of Station H. Rick and I agreed that it was best for me to deal with the logistics—by now the doctors were at least somewhat used to working with me, and Rick's presence tended to confuse the issues. The next morning found me by Ned's bedside in the Otto-Hoffen-Heim, firm in my resolve to bring him home.

The *Ärzte* in evidence were Drs. Vierke and Lützen. They sized me up quickly as they made their rounds and we convened a conference in the privacy of the nurses' station. It began inauspiciously; despite the obvious chairs we all stood and eyed one another warily across the table.

The conversation began with the central institutional problem: Dr. Waldemeyer was Ned's doctor, which meant that the two people with whom I was negotiating did not have the power to decide whether Ned should stay or go. I was clear that in the conversation with Dr. Lützen and me, the *Oberarzt* had said Ned could go at the weekend—we had even discussed the possibility of our going to Munich the following week—but the doctors were not. Looking back I realize the issue might have been one of language—Dr. Lützen's and my conversation with Dr. Waldemeyer had been in English and there might have been some confusion between saying that Ned could go home *for* the weekend and that he could go home *at* or even *by* the weekend. In any case, the two medics who faced me were terrified at the prospect of Dr. Waldemeyer returning from his conference to find Ned gone from Station H.

I explained that I was willing to sign any necessary forms to take him out on my own recognizance. The cornered doctors were equally unwilling to accept this because it suggested their intransigence. We finally compromised on a plan in which Ned would come home on the weekend and return to see Dr. Waldemeyer at seven-forty-five the following Monday, February 12.

But even as we reached this decision, it became clear that the specific date on which Ned left the hospital was not really the issue. The deeper issue was whether the hospital and its doctors had taken good care of him. It was not something I had brought up. Nor did I want to discuss it. I had assiduously avoided making complaints, including any mention of Dieter's performance the night before. Nonetheless, the question of Ned's treatment hung heavy in the air of the nurses' station. Finally, at some point in the wrangling about whether Ned could get adequate care with outpatient physical therapy and home support, Dr. Lützen put in a comment that marked a turn in the tide: "We are not perfect," he said, "but we have done the best we could."

"No," I said, "you aren't perfect. I'm not perfect either. None of us is. But it is time for Ned to come home."

"But his arm does not move very well," the doctor insisted.

"No," I agreed, "but do you have any way to make it move better? For weeks Ned has sat on a bed while we have tried to move this arm; he has been told to sit for hours flexing his elbow through pain, fever, and alienation. He has suffered terribly and it has not worked. His arm is still very stiff. We will continue to try to move it when he is at home. We will come to physical therapy, he will wear his splints, I will play ball with him, he will exercise his fingers on the clarinet, we will move it in any way we can. And maybe it will get better."

The tension in the room was palpable. I did not seem able to defend my ability to take care of Ned at home without seeming critical to the doctors. "Or maybe it won't," I continued doggedly. "Maybe, as your Chief so kindly told me, Ned will always be *behindert*. That is very hard for you to consider, because you are doctors and it is your job to make Ned better. But, you must see that it is equally hard for me to consider, because I am his mother and he is my child. But that does not change the situation. And it makes it all the more true that he should go home. Ned has to begin to live again."

Somehow this was the right thing to say. The clearly defined elbow as pictured and measured by X ray and *Winkelmesser* did not provide us common ground for our discussion. On the contrary, it was the basis of a rigid distinction between them as experts and me as a layperson. It was instead an embodied elbow that provided us with a common ground; an elbow that was attached to Ned who was sitting in a bed across the hall struggling to come to terms with all that had happened to him since a fall in a school playground six month before. Appropriate responses to this elbow were not clear and discrete black balls among a host of whites. They were purely relative; the doctors and I were defining them as we called from barge to shore across the table.

Dr. Vierke volunteered to call outpatient physical therapy, while Dr. Lützen filled out the forms. Left without a task, I propped my shoe on the edge of the table to tie it. Two sets of German eyebrows went up and I realized how gauche I was being.

"*Ich bin Amerikanerin,* I am an American." I offered apologetically. "That's true!" the doctors laughed back.

That afternoon, when Rick, Ned, and I walked into the Villa Walther Ned's cheery chalk murals had long since been washed away, and the cherubs supported their balcony with elbows bent at angles he could no longer attain. But the wispy little boy did not notice. "Can we light candles for dinner?"

Ned and Brady played *Magic* on the floor of the living room, Rick read a book, and I cooked supper. Ned set the table, and lit the candles. We all sat and ate together. Brady did the dishes. Rick read to Ned. I sat and listened too.

On Saturday evening Matteus came over with a fistful of fireworks to celebrate Ned's homecoming. The American in me cringed, but from Ned's perspective legal fireworks were one of the real perks of German life. The boys went to the fish pond behind the Villa Walther to light them. Brady watched from the reserved distance of the second-floor balcony. After the first bang, Christopher emerged with the twins who jumped and squealed Roo-like at his knees. A "jumping jack" whirled, fizzed, and changed colors. Another cracker banged. The sociologist exploded from his apartment.

"Have you no respect!" he bellowed. His choice of language left no doubt as to whom he held responsible for the disturbance. The observers faded, leaving the boys to deal with his wrath.

On Monday we met the doctor in an unfamiliar room in the surgical wing of the hospital. As he worked Ned's arm on the table I asked whether we had made a mistake to taper the morphine so quickly, whether we had been wrong to take him home. "His angles were so good at the beginning of last week," I ventured. "Shouldn't we put him back on painkillers to keep them that way? I would let him go back to the hospital if he had to, in order to be on morphine."

"He can't be on painkillers forever," Dr. Waldemeyer said. "He must sometime move it by himself."

"Yes," I responded, "but not necessarily this week. Shouldn't we give it a try?"

"No." The surgeon was firm. "He must move it by himself." He turned to Ned and delivered his now-familiar speech: "Ned, you must move the arm. It is very important. You must move it and move it and move it. I cannot do it for you. Your mother cannot do it for you. It is your arm and you must move it." Ned grinned at me with his recognition of this formula as we got up to go.

I fussed to Rick, but he did not want to enter my tightly focused world of daily angle measures. "Ned's home and in physical therapy. His arm is crooked, but it was in the hospital too. Let it lie, Joan!" I did my best. After all, it was I who had brought Ned home.

While I battled my abstract demons, Ned and Rick battled mundane ones. In our division of the medical territory I talked to doctors but Rick was in charge of physical therapy. Ned had physical therapy twice a day. This meant that even though he was at home his life was completely dominated by the Otto-Hoffen-Heim. I kept hoping for some dramatic improvement, but Ned just wanted to stop. He had had enough of this whole performance, and fiercely resented the relentless schedule of outpatient care. "I missed one week of vacation because I was on Station H. Now I'm missing another one because of physical therapy!"

The weather was beastly—too raw and gray to encourage walking but just warm enough to make the ice on top of the deeply frozen *Seen* mushy and unskatable. With Rick there and the boys on vacation, the apartment seemed impossibly crowded. We were all always underfoot, and none of us could think of fun things to do.

"Let's go to the Pergamon Museum, Joan. We didn't make it over Christmas and everyone says it's lovely."

"But it's all the way across town. If we leave right now we'd get there between eleven-thirty and twelve. Ned's physical therapy is at three, so we'd have to be back by two-fifteen to catch the 2:43 bus. We'd be there only an hour! It doesn't seem worth it." I struggled to be constructive. "But we could try the Dahlem Museum. It's on the way to the Otto-Hoffen-Heim."

Rick, too, tried to be upbeat. "Sure. Come on, Ned. We are going to the Dahlem Museum!"

"No, I hate museums."

"Well, then. Why don't you go to physical therapy on your own?"

"NO! You promised you'd take me to physical therapy. I hate physical therapy. If you don't take me, I won't go!"

"OK, Ned." Rick had had it. "But I didn't promise I would not take you to a museum beforehand."

Ned sat on a bench in the museum resolutely staring at a wall while Rick and I walked through the European gallery. We saw the pictures and afterwards Ned had Rick's company for physical therapy. No one felt fulfilled.

* * *

At our next appointment with Dr. Waldemeyer during his regular Wednesday office hours, there was a sense of quiet helplessness. Ned's arm was, if anything, stiffer than it had been on Monday. "He goes to physical therapy?" the doctor asked sadly. When I answered in the affirmative, he just sighed and said: "Come back next week."

I got home miserable, and Rick suggested that I call Dr. Lyman. It made sense. Of course it was important to get another opinion. But even as I did the sensible thing I realized how truly I had moved to Berlin. I saw that when it came to Ned's elbow I no longer believed that Dr. Lyman was intrinsically more to be trusted than Dr. Waldemeyer. I saw no reason to believe that a doctor in America would know more, could do more, than had already been done.

Still, I called Dr. Lyman and once again brought the Providence pediatrician up to date on Ned's situation. "This all seems a bit complicated," he said. "I'd better call an orthopedic surgeon."

Two days later Dr. Lyman called back. Instead of the cheerful reassurance we had been looking for, he was grave. "My consultant said the situation is very serious," he said. "He wants to see Ned's arm."

I panicked. How could I send Ned to America now? He was not in school there. Rick could not deal with him from work. I would have to go too. What would happen to Brady? Besides I had meant it when I said that Ned had to begin to live again. I could not let him be drawn into another drama of heroic attempts to fix his elbow.

"What if we sent the file?" I offered. "If I sent all of the X rays, MRIs, and operation reports from Dr. Waldemeyer, wouldn't that be good enough?"

"Oh!" Dr. Lyman replied. "That would be even better! But they are central to Ned's file. Dr. Waldemeyer might not want to send them."

"Let me try," I said.

I hung up, momentarily triumphant because I had avoided, at least temporarily, moving the story to a whole new level of complexity. But as I set about calling Dr. Waldemeyer to ask for Ned's files, I felt like a traitor. I knew he had done his level best and I did not doubt his work. Still, determined, I left my message on his machine. On Sunday night the surgeon called me back.

"Hello, Mrs. Richards. You asked for me?"

What to say? "I called Dr. Lyman," I admitted, "and his orthopedic consultant said he wants to see Ned."

"What?" Dr. Waldemeyer asked. "Whatever for?"

"I guess he thinks that something else might be done about the elbow," I explained. "I don't think anyone but you, Ned, and I has any idea of how much has already been done or of how frustrating a left elbow can be."

"I guess not," Dr. Waldemeyer admitted wryly. "Maybe we need more. When do you send him?"

"I told Dr. Lyman I did not want to send him, that I would send the pictures instead. I need the X rays, the MRIs, and the operation reports."

"Of course," he said. "We get them for you tomorrow. But I do not think that he will find anything. I think the situation is completely normal. I was thinking about it the other night," he went on, musing. "I do not think that what Ned is doing is unusual. He does not seem to me to be angry or depressed. Sometimes he is interested in his arm and then he works on it; sometimes he is not, and then he doesn't. My son would be the same."

I hung up, comforted, but also a little guilty. Dr. Waldemeyer saw what I did, that the X rays and MRIs had very little to say about Ned's elbow movement. I had no doubt that the pictures were "normal" as he put it; for just this reason they were obviously no substitute for Ned whose elbow was so clearly *not* normal. Leibniz whispered in my ear: "For space denotes an order to things which exist at the same time, considered as existing together. . . . And when many things are seen together one perceives that order of things among themselves." And when many things are not seen together there is no order to perceive. Ned's X rays told very little about Ned's elbow. There was much more to the situation than that.

"Joan, where's Ned's Dynasplint?"

"I don't know. Didn't you take it to physical therapy yesterday?"

"Yes. But I've looked everywhere and I can't find it."

"You lost the Dynasplint! It is important! Ned is supposed to wear it for half an hour after physical therapy!"

"I know! That's why I'm looking for it!"

"Damn it, Rick! It cost almost 3,000 marks!"

Rick had left the Dynasplint at the bank but it took us four anger-filled days to locate it. On Tuesday he flew home with Ned's medical file, frustrated and exhausted. He was coming again in April and we would try again then. For the moment, though, we lived in two different places and it mattered.

The lonely week waiting for Dr. Lyman's response to Ned's file was excruciating. The seminar that week focused on quantum mechanics and generated a luncheon discussion about the ultimate viability of objective knowledge.

"The issue really comes down to the communication of information. In the subatomic realm it is simply impossible to create an image because of the interaction between the photons and the things being pictured."

"What happens if you get less theoretical? Let's look at the X rays of Ned's elbow. Or at his angle measures. Both are objective images, but I am not at all clear about the relationship between image and reality, symbol and truth, in his case."

"Oh! Is your son back from the hospital? How does it go with his arm?"

They were being kind, but I had not asked in order to garner sympathy. Mine were pressing questions, and I wanted help in thinking about them.

At Thursday night's dinner I talked over the situation with one of the fellow's wives.

"You should go to Boston," she said firmly. "Of course you should go at once!"

"But how could I do that? It is too much time already. I have to do my work sometime!" I objected.

"Your work is very important," she said. "But your child is more important. You should take him to Boston Children's Hospital. If they cannot fix the elbow, you should take him to the Mayo Clinic. You must do everything for him: nothing else matters."

I didn't know how to respond. Of course Ned's elbow was important, but other things *did* matter. Did my work and I have no place at all?

I asked the woman: "But what about your husband? Would he give up this fellowship year to take care of one of your children's elbow?"

"No, he wouldn't," she said. "He is not their mother. But he would give up anything to go to war if it was called for. Men give up their work all the time for things that are centrally important. And no one blames or penalizes them for it."

"Yes, they come home to the GI bill," I said.

"So you must go, too," she said. "Your work will wait."

I knew that my work would not wait. Every day was a day lost and I could do nothing about it. I explained that I had sent the pictures to Boston and they were deciding what should be done.

✻ ✻ ✻

The next day Dr. Lyman called back. "My orthopedic advisor looked at the pictures. He says you have done what you can for the moment. He said that in many ways Americans have a great deal to learn from the Germans. It is very important that Ned keep up with his physical therapy. But the last thing he needs right now is more surgery."

Niederlage (Failure)

So Ned was out of the hospital and the doctors were in agreement that enough had been done. February vacation was over, and he was back in school. Brady was back in school. Rick was back at work. I also should have been at work, but I was not. I was desperate. For a few weeks I had let the Otto-Hoffen-Heim give me the order that had been destroyed in me. But now even the direction afforded by day-to-day crisis and commitment was gone. I couldn't work. I couldn't think.

Night after night I could not sleep; I began to taking advantage of the time warp of distance. Depending on which coast you call, at three o'clock in the morning in Berlin it is either six or nine in the evening in the United States. I made calls in my dark nights. It was a blessed relief to find company then, though my American friends did not understand the circumstances in which I found myself.

"It's Ned's left arm? But he's right-handed! It doesn't really matter, does it?" *I'd like to hear you say that about your child!*

"Joan! It must be two-thirty in the morning where you are. You must be depressed if you are having such trouble sleeping." *Yes, and what do you suggest I do about it? Ask Dr. Waldemeyer for Prozac?*

I kept my sharp comments to myself and listened eagerly to their familiar voices. The comfort of the calls was often enough to buy me an hour or two of sleep.

At least once a week Genie and I had breakfast together. We had finally fixed on the perfect place, a patisserie that opened at seven-thirty and was both within walking distance of the Villa Walther and on her way to work. There we nibbled croissants, sipped *milch Kafe* [café latte], and talked. We talked about everything: about our children; about probability, certainty, and necessity; about differences in the intellectual worlds of the eighteenth and nineteenth centuries; about German views of hierarchy and responsibility. By the time we were through, I would have some sense of clarity, but I could not hold it. By the time I got back to the *Kolleg* the world was murky again.

It was not easy for me to go to the *Wissenschaftskolleg* at all. The little office that had been so warm and sunny in the fall was cold and dark in February. The place that had once held out such hope to me had come to represent professional failure. A book requires time to come together, to develop. Time was just what I had come to Berlin to find, and Ned's elbow had stolen it. In the more than six months since we had come to Berlin it seemed I had spent less time in my office than in any other place; the hospital, the 110 bus, even trips to the grocery store probably accounted for more hours of my German time. The very air in my office reproached me.

Lunches continued, relentlessly elegant, their formality a daily reminder of how poorly my inner life coincided with the world I was supposed to be inhabiting. I tried to live up to the expectations they represented, to eat what was put before me, to be gracious to whomever might sit beside me, to seem intelligent. But I found it a struggle to be polite, always a guest at someone else's table.

I fared better at breakfast, which was an unofficial meal. Starting at eight a ragtag combination of fellows would straggle in for rolls, cereal, or leftovers. Some sat alone, others congregated at a central table. Conversation, if there was any, was relaxed, and informal. I sipped my coffee and reveled in the unexpected freedom of a German breakfast where you can eat whatever you like: salad, pepper salami, cheese, yesterday's casserole.

German class was dwindling as fellows became frustrated with the glacially slow process of learning another language. "It's just a waste of time. I'm only here for one year. I can't learn it now." But I went doggedly back. Every word learned, every construction mastered, might help me follow what was going on around me, at lunch, in the hospital, at a reception, or in the next seminar.

Besides, when all else failed, German gave me something to focus on. "*Ned läuft in* DIE *Schule.* Ned runs in[to] the school." Boundary crossed, accusative object. "*Ned läuft in* DER *Schule.* Ned runs in[side] the school." Boundary respected, dative object. "*Frau Sonntag* HAT *den elbogen bewegt.* Frau Sonntag moved the elbow." Transitive verb, action on an object. "*Ned* HAT *den elbogen* BEWEGT. Ned moved the elbow." Transitive verb, action on an object. "*Der elbogen* HAT BEWOGEN. The elbow moved." Intransitive verb, action contained by object. While walking for groceries, preparing meals, or straightening the apartment I repeated such sentences over and over trying to make them come naturally. At the same time, I mused on the unfamiliar distinctions, their world of crisply delineated insides and outsides.

Non-German speakers began to cut the seminars given in German. "The speakers are your colleagues and they deserve your attention," the permanent fellows scolded. The response was mixed: "I came here to get my work done. It is simply stupid for me to spend two hours sitting listening to a seminar and discussion in a language I cannot understand. I will only go to seminars in English!"

"But they come to our seminars. They've given us a whole year of support. It's little enough to ask."

"I don't mind. I bring a problem with me and think it out during seminar."

I continued to attend absolutely faithfully. It was not a particularly illuminating exercise, though. I have never before been a doodler, but now my note pages were covered with inexpert drawings. My German was improving, I understood more, and I kept trying to formulate constructive questions. Unbidden, others appeared on my pad as well: "What does this have to do with *anything*?" I asked neither the constructive nor the nonconstructive ones. They lay on the page entwined in vines or lodged in exploding volcanoes.

The clearest thing in life was Ned's arm, and I didn't understand what was happening with it. I needed to talk to Dr. Waldemeyer. I didn't know where to begin with my questions, but I knew that I needed him to help me understand.

At first I looked forward to our appointments because I thought that there we could talk together, but they were not conducive to conversation. They took place all over the hospital before whatever audience engaged the surgeon at the moment of our arrival.

"One hundred twenty degrees of flexion? I don't think so. It looks like a hundred to me. Do you wear your bending splint?"

"Yes."

"Do you bend your arm in school?"

"I try to."

"Try leaning on it when you can. Like this." The doctor demonstrated leaning with bent elbow against a wall. "Lean on it at your desk. Keep bending it. If you keep trying, you can do better than this. This is not good."

He turned to me to make sure I had registered what he was saying.

"He must exercise. After physical therapy he must wear the Dynasplint for half an hour. Then he must exercise—play basketball, go swimming. Then he wears the Dynasplint for an hour. Then he leans on the wall. . . ." My eyes glazed over as he prescribed endless hours of activity in half-hour increments.

The appointments made Ned furious. "You said Germans talk about the elbow. Well, Dr. Waldemeyer doesn't. He's always telling me it's *my* elbow and I have to move it. Well, it *is* my elbow and he's lucky it's not his. I don't move my elbow because it *hurts!*"

He responded with a passive-aggressive sleepiness that was hard for the doctor to understand or me to mediate.

"Sir, you know it doesn't help Ned to tell him it is his elbow and he has to move it. He knows that and he is trying."

"But it's true! It *is* his elbow. And I always like to be encouraging!"

I spoke to a German colleague about the situation in hopes that he could give me some kind of insight into the German medical mind.

"As long as you keep coming back, the case is open. *Er will sich seine Niederlage nicht einstehen.*" More words from the vocabulary sessions of my sleepless nights. *Niederlage:* failure, defeat; *sich einstehen;* face up to, admit. *Er will sich seine Niederlage nicht einstehen;* he does not want to admit his defeat, face up to his failure.

I could not accept this interpretation, and confirmed my hopes in the brief times the surgeon and I spoke to each other directly. Every time I called to set up the next appointment he would eagerly ask about the progress of physical therapy. Surely he wouldn't ask so hopefully if he had given up.

"He's getting stronger, but his angles just stay the same. I *wish* they'd get better, even just a little bit!"

"Oh, Mrs. Richards. I do, too."

He wouldn't say it if it weren't true, I assured myself. And he wouldn't waste his time hoping if the elbow was beyond hope. *Er will sich seine Niederlage nicht einstehen.* My colleague had it all wrong. There must be hope.

Ned

All of my struggles to understand were basically irrelevant to Ned. His problems were immediate, deep, and only incidentally related to his elbow. The third operation and hospitalization had been the final straw for his relationship to Germany, and the air again rang with his wish to go home. I tried my best to stay out of a dynamic that led us into fruitless fights.

"Isn't the *See* beautiful this morning? Look at how still it is . . . and those little ducks! I love this walk to the bus in the morning."

"Providence is beautiful too, Mom."

"Yes it is. I didn't say it wasn't. But I don't think your walk to school is as pretty as this."

"We have the Hope High School field."

"True, but it is not like walking down a path by the water."

"I'd rather have the Hope High School field."

The physical therapists bore the brunt of Ned's anger and his sorrow. He was thoroughly tired of the hospital and fought physical therapy with a will.

I tried to be encouraging but my attempts at cheer were not much more successful than Dr. Waldemeyer's litany about movement. "Physical therapy! Physical therapy! No, Mom. I did not have a good time in physical therapy. It's boring! Why do I have to go? I can't play with anyone after school because I go to dumb old physical therapy. That's why I don't have any friends!"

I tried to help Ned with his friends. When he first arrived in the fall, he had quickly and effectively created a niche for himself among the children in his class. Within three months of the initial contact, however, it was effectively broken, by hospitalizations, physical therapies, and major vacations in December and February. From the first of December until the end of a two-week February vacation, Ned was in school only sporadically and even then only for truncated days. His first-term report card noted twenty-three days plus twenty-seven hours absent.

Ned's first day back was February 19, which was also his birthday. In our minds' eyes both he and I had anticipated a hero's return; what he faced in fact was no response at all. "They are used to me being gone," he reported sadly. "They forget to ask me to sit with them and then there is no room at the table." I tried to help by inviting several children for a birthday party at home. Still it was several weeks before he was comfortable in school again.

Readjusting to school was a step in the right direction but there was more to Ned's problem than that. While I was taking him literally and focusing on his school friends, he was struggling with a broken heart. For the entire four weeks on Station H Petra and Ned had delighted in each other. Petra listened to Ned, she acted as his advocate with the nurses, she counseled him in his attempts to relate to his German room-mates. She laughed with him at the strange world of German television, of Station H, of multilingual negotiation. She stayed with him through his pain, his tears, his infection, his temper. She gave everything to Ned. He loved her and let her move his arm.

When I took Ned out of the hospital, Petra was gone. He still had physical therapy, but now it was with the outpatient department. Petra was an inpatient physical therapist and he could not work with her any more. I had thought Ned was weak and tired, and he was. There was also an unspoken issue, however; Ned wanted to go back to Petra.

For Ned's birthday Petra sent him a T-shirt she had decorated with *"Calimero mit Sombrero."* The next day Ned's school German class was on television as some kind of human-interest short. "I was wearing Petra's T-shirt, Mom! So when she is watching the news she will see me and she will see the shirt. Do you think it will show up? so she knows I'm wearing it?"

"I'm sure she will, dear. How was physical therapy today?"

"Oh, it was OK, I guess."

I was too focused on his angles to realize why Ned was so miserable as an outpatient. But one day while we were waiting for Dr. Walde-meyer, Petra came through with one of her colleagues.

"Hey, Ned!" she whooped.

"Hey, Petra! What do you do to your shoe?"

"I *buckle* it," she said, using the vocabulary he had taught her to refer to her Birkenstocks.

They beamed at each other and fell silent, their interchange stran-gled by the public gaze of the waiting room.

"Well! I see you, Ned!" she said finally.

"I will see you, Petra!" he said, carefully emphasizing the future tense.

Dear Petra,

I am writing to thank you for all you have done for Ned. I realize he was the first patient of your career and you did a beautiful job with him.

I know that you have worked professionally with Ned. At the same time, you became his friend. He misses you terribly and would very much like to see you again. I do not know how physical therapists handle this kind of thing, and will accept whatever you think is best. But I do want to give you permission to see him, if you like. Perhaps you could have a cup of cocoa with him in the cafeteria after his physical therapy and your workday, or some sunny day you might take a walk with him through the *Naturschutzgebiet,* or you might just call him some evening at 555 18 81; he would love to talk with you.

In any case, you have been a wonderful friend and physical therapist to him and I want to thank you.

Sincerely yours,
Joan L Richards

Petra did not take Ned to cocoa nor walk with him in the *Naturschutzge-biet.* Instead, on the day she received my note, she and her boyfriend invited Ned, Brady, and me to dinner on a Saturday night. Petra's boyfriend prepared fondue, and we cooked our little pieces of meat and vegetables late into the night. The evening eased Ned's pain; he saw that Petra was still his friend and was comforted.

With this development, after-school physical therapy began to get better. The casualty of the adjustment was Sigrid, whose youth and English had recommended her before Christmas. Ned's grumpiness was simply too much for the brisk young woman and she was slowly replaced in Ned's world by Frau Sonntag. Frau Sonntag was from former East Germany, which meant that she spoke little to no English. On the other hand, she was the mother of grown sons. She had several times lived with someone of Ned's ilk and had the patience to deal with his sorrows. As the winter moved slowly into spring she played with him, hugged him, and ruffled his hair. He began to perk up.

Frau Sonntag's formula for Ned's sessions was energetic. *"Fünf Minuten strecken, fünf Minuten beugen, und zwanzig Minuten* SPIELEN!" [Five minutes of stretching, five minutes of bending, and twenty minutes of GAMES!"] Ned became a mountain climber who belayed from runged walls on ropes; he became a racer lying face down on a little cart and propelling himself with his arms; he became a left-handed tennis player hitting heavy balls over an imaginary net with a bowling pin. *"Wir spielen nicht wie* BABIES!" [We don't play like BABIES!"], Frau Sonntag would cry as she whammed a huge, heavy red ball at Ned with her bowling pin. Ned would cry *"Nicht Babies!"* as he hit it back to her side of the room with his.

Often Ned's afternoon session was the last of the day, and the half hour would stretch to three-quarters of an hour or more. As their days wound down, others would join in and the competition would mount. Ned would come home triumphant, having beaten a physical therapy student in a cart race or been on a winning doubles team in "tennis." He stopped complaining about physical therapy.

In the process of getting Ned out of the hospital, I had insisted to all and sundry that I could stay on top of his needs at home. This was not a trivial assignment. In February and March, Berlin warmed up, but not much. The sky remained dark and gray, the air damp and chill, the *Seen* lifeless and black under their cover of mushy ice. Day after day I pushed Ned into the raw afternoons to play made-up ball games. When our energy and/or patience gave out, we would carry groceries in bags hanging from our left arms.

Some of my efforts were directed toward identifying after-school programs in which Ned could participate, but here I was doomed to failure. The doctor kept harping on basketball as excellent therapy, but I could not identify a single public court in which we could carry out the man's repeated directives that we play. The school team's season had begun when Ned was in some stage of casted life; at this point it was moving toward its climax, and there was no room for a newcomer with a weak and crooked left arm. So except for occasional pathetic attempts at a flimsy portable hoop rigged up on a trestled gate of the Villa Walther we had to shelve the basketball suggestion.

I worked out a scheme in which Beth would take Ned swimming with the twins. In the event, all the goodwill in the world could not maintain this as a regular program across the disparity in their ages. However, the times they did go showed that Ned could still navigate well in the water. So I decided to push harder on the idea and called the coach of the team he had joined in the fall. I explained that Ned would not be able to swim as fast as the rest of the team, but that he would improve quickly and would practice eagerly.

She was firm and clear. "I am committed to competitive swimming," she explained. "It sounds terrible. I don't like to say it, but I just do not have the time to work with someone like your son who has no chance of winning in any event."

That week the seminar at the *Wissenschaftskolleg* was about the voyage of a sixteenth-century slave ship. It was in English so I could relax as I listened. "O God. Thy sea is so big and my boat is so small," appeared on my notepad. Don't be so melodramatic, Joan, I admonished myself. But without my really intending it, the paper produced a picture: my little sailboat with a broken mast, adrift in a world of wiggly waves. How was I going to get used to this? How was I going to help Ned through this?

Over time, all of my somewhat forced attempts to work Ned's arm faded to be replaced by more natural ones. "Foursquare" was the first sport in which Ned began to make his comeback. This simple game where four participants bounce a ball back and forth was the major recess activity among the boys in his class and he attempted it with a will. About three weeks after he had returned to school he announced triumphantly: "I made King in foursquare today."

"Good deal! Does that happen a lot?"

"No, Mom! Don't be silly! I have never made King since I got back from the hospital. It's hard to play foursquare with a broken arm."

The other initially risky but ultimately successful program was baseball. Early in March I bravely asked Rick to supply mitts, so that Ned and I could play catch. I did not know what to expect the first time we went out. There was even some question as to whether Ned could hold his fingers straight enough to get the mitt onto his left hand. He managed, though, and out we went to throw balls back and forth in the rose garden behind the Villa Walther. The experiment was a success. Ned had a significantly reduced reach, but he was still a very good catch, and his throwing was as good as ever. In fact the only problem with the exercise was my reluctance to catch balls thrown as hard as Ned was wont to throw his. I rejoiced as proper spring approached and a regular baseball team was organized at Ned's school.

On Friday, April 4, Rick arrived for his last visit to Germany. Ned's medical mess had rendered his previous visit so disastrous that this time we were determined to escape the whole scene. We firmly told all and sundry at the Otto-Hoffen-Heim that we were going to Munich for the week. Early on Saturday morning we left under a clutter of baggage and more—the boys brought skis, poles, and ski boots. If the weather held, it was possible we could find some spring skiing. We would be staying in a tiny pied à terre Genie's husband had in Munich, which was empty because their family was away on vacation. It was the first time Brady, Ned, or I had been out of Berlin since August; we were taking the fast train.

No sooner did we leave Berlin than Ned got a flu. He stayed feverish in bed for the first couple of days of the visit and Brady was engaged in an English term paper that was stubbornly expanding to fill the time allotted. It was not what Rick and I had planned, but we were getting used to that, and their being housebound left us free to explore the new city. On Munich's neutral ground we could be together again.

Tuesday afternoon, when Rick and I came back from a long exploratory walk we found Ned's bed empty. We could hear muffled rhythmic chanting through the bathroom door.

"What are you singing, Ned?"

"Oh, nothing!" Ned emerged, newly cleaned and clad in his *Schlafanzug,* the German pajamas I'd bought under nurse's orders.

"Oh, come on! Tell us!"

Ned grinned wickedly. He extended his arms to look cool, and began a rhythmic shuffle to the rap of the song he'd made up from German phrases encountered in gym classes. His *Schlafanzug* began to sag.

Mr. Rap hat gesagt: Ja! Ja!	Mr. Rap said: Yes! Yes!
Mr. Rap hat gesagt: Ja! Ja!	Mr. Rap said: Yes! Yes!
Setz dich!	Sit down!
Steh auf!	Stand up!
Geh raus!	Go out!
Setz dich!	Sit down!
Steh auf!	Stand up!
Geh raus!	Go out!

He returned to the chorus more quietly to regain his breath:

Mr. Rap hat gesagt: Ja! Ja!	Mr. Rap said: Yes! Yes!
Mr. Rap hat gesagt: Ja! Ja!	Mr. Rap said: Yes! Yes!

Then, again loud.

Auf die Plätze!	On your marks
Fertig!	Get set!

Los!	Go!
Auf die Plätze!	On your marks!
Fertig!	Get set!
Los!	Go!

And again the chorus:

Mr. Rap hat gesagt: Ja! Ja!	Mr. Rap said: Yes! Yes!
Mr. Rap hat gesagt: Ja! Ja!	Mr. Rap said: Yes! Yes!

Brady protested: "Mom! Dad! Stop him! He's being so stupid!"

But Rick and I didn't stop him. We were laughing as we hadn't laughed in months.

When Ned's flu had subsided, Rick and I took the boys skiing. We rose early, caught the train to Garmisch-Partenkirchen and then the cog railway up and through the Zugspitze, the highest mountain in Germany. The weather was not good—the peak was totally engulfed in fog—but that just meant that I could not see enough to be terrified in the gondola on the way down. It certainly didn't bother the boys, who skied happily, Brady's lanky form leading the way, Ned's indescribable hat flapping in the wind behind. Rick and I enjoyed ourselves together, watching our children and the German lodge crowd.

In our absence the *Seen* thawed. As we schlepped skis and luggage back to the apartment on Saturday, their waters moved and sparkled in the afternoon's light.

England

4/16/96

Dear Joan,

The flight home was uneventful. Apparently there was a 6" snowstorm last Wednesday but now it is almost all gone except for piles lurking in sunless corners of parking lots. Daffodils blooming in the backyard. It just needs a little attention to be ready to take off. The major project is preparing Ned's garden, which means burying the compost pile in it. That's actually a little work, but really the only major thing. Give the boys my love and tell Brady if he is going to spend every waking hour on the computer he might as well send e-mail to his Dad!

"Bro! Dude! Want to play Monopoly?"

"Outta here, Ned! Marina and I are studying for our history exam!"

The sun reflected off the *See* into twinkling patterns on our living room ceiling. After school, after physical therapy, rebuffed by his brother, Ned sprawled on the squooshy couch, bored and lazy. "Go on out!" I commanded. "Do something! Go row the boat!" Even as the words popped out of my mouth I realized I was sending him on a fool's errand but Ned leapt at the suggestion. He shared none of my doubts as he carried the oars, one in each hand, down to the boathouse grotto. He had equally few doubts when he carried them back, an hour later, having rowed to the end of the linked chain of *Seen* and back.

"Know what? I can row you to the grocery store, Mom!"

It was a slow trip. The boat did not always go straight and Ned was not very strong. But for several days he rowed me about half a mile to get milk, pasta, and eggs. I sat in the bow and watched him very closely—it seemed extraordinary that he could do it at all. But each day he got better, our passage smoother, the trip through the *Seen* more beautiful.

Brady was on a class trip for the last two weeks of April, and Ned's medical situation seemed all too stable. So I arranged for him to stay with Sean, who lived close enough to the Otto-Hoffen-Heim that he could walk to physical therapy. Petra volunteered to take him to his required appointments with Dr. Waldemeyer. I then flew to England. I had to begin getting organized for my seminar at the beginning of June. At the Dibner I had worked on De Morgan's probability theory. At the *Wissenschaftskolleg* I would follow his next step into logic, but I hadn't worked on this aspect of his work before. I could use a couple of weeks rummaging in the archives. In any case, I had to get out of Berlin. I needed some distance; I needed to take stock.

In England I stayed in De Morgan's London, in Bloomsbury, and I passed his collegial descendants on my way to and from the various archives that housed his papers. They walked briskly down Gower Street, as he had once done, carrying their briefcases, minds on their next appointment. I thought of a piece of doggerel De Morgan had once written while Sophia and the children were vacationing in Marathon.

> The Mountains look on Marathon
> And Marathon looks on the sea
> All very fine to look upon
> But what the deuce is that to me!

These men's families were probably not in Marathon, but they were elsewhere.

So was mine, I reminded myself. Now I too could control my time. But still I found it hard to concentrate. I was acutely aware that none of my English mathematicians, not Newton, not De Morgan, not Ellis, would have allowed a woman, certainly not a mother, into the sanctity of their mathematical world. For years I had acknowledged their position and taken pride in showing them to be wrong. I had organized and controlled my life as ably as they; I had entered their colleges and their mathematical world as an equal.

In London I tried to reestablish my place in the mathematical world that for so long had been my solace and support, but I could not. There was still plenty of material for me to work on, but I was no longer comfortable with it. My sabbatical time as Ned's mother had left its mark. I was there under false pretenses, an impostor, an intruder. I constantly felt De Morgan's judgment of me as a woman working in a man's world, and as I read his letters I found myself judging him in return.

March 8,1844

My dear Sir John,

[Insurance] Tables A and B shall be put in hand forthwith, and I dare say you will have them at the end of next week. . . . But who knows anything about such young children's lives. Table makers put them down as in duty bound—but for any use children's lives are of before seven, you might just as well substitute young puppies, and insure human children upon an average of *them*. . . . Children of that age will no more stand quiet to be tabulated than to have their hair brushed. . . .

I thought of Alice, who was turning six that June, and thus more than a year from her father's border between puppy and human. I couldn't help noting the difference between Augustus's and Sophia's description of their child.

December 25, 1843

My dear Sir John,

I send you the complements of the season in the shape of two formulae, fattened expressly for Christmas, or at least expanded, which is all one. . . .

I saw Augustus writing in his quiet study as the smells of a roasting bird wafted under the closed door. Outside Sophia juggled children, servants, and a real meal. I doubted that for her a fattened bird and an expanded equation seemed "all one."

I found myself thinking on the words of Caroline of Ansbach: "Philosophy was made, or ought to be sought, in order to make us more tranquil in spirit and to strengthen us against ourselves and against everything outside us which may assail us." The kind of professional mathematics that De Morgan was in the process of developing seemed to reach toward her tranquil ideal by isolating its practitioners rather than by strengthening them.

Certainly it did not strengthen me against myself or against those things that were assailing me. The more I read, the grumpier and less productive I became. I was glad when the end of the week meant I could go to Cambridge. I knew a number of historians of science there. It would be fun to talk to them.

But when I got to Cambridge I realized I had become a social liability who would drown anyone who asked even the most innocuous question under torrents of words. "Your son broke his left elbow?" Simply saying "yes" won't explain anything. "But why didn't you just send him home?" Even were this the way I handled problems, when in the process would I have simply sent him home? "But surely there was time between the operations?" How to explain the time of convalescence and of healing? That was elbow time, physical therapy time, mother time— "*Know what? I can row you to the grocery store, Mom!*" That was purely relative time; for Frau Professor Doktor Richards inexplicably wasted time. If I once set out to explain myself, I would go on for hours. I was staying with friends who were kind, but after a couple of slips, I stayed away from everyone else.

In the archives my troubles continued. "On the absolute substantive *reality* of all the primary truths of mathematics I have never had any doubt: but I have an idea that different people hold them by different hooks," De Morgan wrote in 1844. His liberal attitude was all very well, but I couldn't find any hook. I agreed with Ellis, who wrote to a friend: "I doubt if a man of mind so active as yours and so capable of various exertions can quite understand the nuisance it is to me to struggle day by day with mere abstractions. . . ." I was not like Ellis in being sick or "faint for lack of breakfast and pinched with cold," but I certainly understood that the press of experience could make it difficult to maintain interest in the minutiae of the mathematical structures through which we define certainty, probability, and knowledge.

Disengaged though I was, I realized it would be silly not to finish the one real box of De Morgan in the Whewell correspondence. I held myself still and kept reading.

My Dear Sir,

. . . A pupil of mine had been colouring maps—with of course a different colour for all countries which have common boundary line. . . . He found that he never had occasion to use more than *four* colours—and that he could not make a case in which more than four would be wanted—

It was a find! I had never seen this particular presentation of the four-color problem and in this letter, which went on for pages, De Morgan was linking his thinking about it to logical issues. I read it carefully to the end:

Yours truly,
Augustus De Morgan
7 Camden Town
Dec 9, 1853

I stopped short. "*Her father did not realise the degree of illness till the end was near and the blow fell heavily upon him.*" The letter was written just two weeks before Alice died. I hated it.

*   *   *

I returned to the archives only briefly to get a microfilm of the De Morgan material sent to me at the *Wissenschaftskolleg*. For the rest of the week I wandered through the museums, parks, and streets of Cambridge, keeping to myself as much as possible. Around and above me the city's towers pointed spired gables or reached with open palms to God and transcendent truth. But I was not viewing the city from a postcard's distance. I was in its midst, and what I saw was walls.

Walls divided the colleges from the surrounding city; more walls divided each college from its neighbors; yet another set divided areas within the colleges, fellows from students, students from visitors. Outside the streets were full of people, of commerce and of tourists who flocked around huge buses. Schoolchildren walked to and fro with book bags; teenagers whooped and giggled in energetic masses; toddlers in strollers rattled by, kicking their feet as mothers chatted above their heads. Inside it was quiet and Newton reigned.

Absolute, true mathematical time . . . Whose time? A doctor's? A mother's? A child's? An elbow's? *Absolute space remains always similar and immovable. . . .* For whom is it useful to think of reality in these terms? *Positions properly have no quantity.* Pictures of Ned's elbow were readily transportable as if positions had no quantity, but were they real? Did they tell the story?

The more I pondered these questions, the more I saw my mathematicians trying to grab the truth, to control it by knowing it. I saw them engaged in a powerful purifying project, trying always to separate the necessary and absolutely true from the contingent and the relative. I had long been intrigued by their effort, but my years with Ned had shown me the dark side of their drive toward purity. Their mathematical work was magnificent, but they had only been able to sustain it by disparaging the relative and consigning it to their servants and their wives. Wives are, after all, merely relative. So, I realized, are mothers. "Ah yes, you are his mother." *"Ich spreche mit der Mutter von einem Kind."* I had lived Ned's medical challenge in relativity, but it had not been a merely pale reflection of an absolute. It had been intensely real.

I sought out Newton, whose statue is seated in a high-windowed hall of Trinity College, and asked him to explain why he had isolated and sanctified absolute time and space. *"Space is the sensorium of God,"* he said. "But," I found myself objecting, "that's just a projection! *God does not stand in need of any organ to perceive things by.*" I stood sadly in front of the unmoving figure. Newton's mathematical world was as lovely as ever but I no longer had a place in it. The gap between Frau Doktor Professor Richards and Ned's mother had closed.

Frühling (Spring)

Ned, Brady and I were reunited in May. True spring, with flowers, bird-song and occasional blue-sky days had finally come to the city. Egg-yolk ducklings paddled behind their mothers; a pair of nesting swans settled on the small island of our little *See*; an individualistic muscovy duck habitually perched about six meters off the ground on top of the obelisk in the back garden. One morning, Ned and I noticed a field mouse cowering by the path as the sociologist's cat approached. "Don't worry!" her owner said as he scooped the predator up. "I make sure she does not kill anything."

In the Villa Walther life became lighter. The twins' chirping joined with that of Berlin's many birds. The English philosopher's family joined him; the arrival of his two children meant there would be more friends for Ned and babysitting jobs for Brady. Games of hide and seek and *tig*, the English word for tag, materialized in the lengthening afternoons.

The fellows had been together for some time. The composition of luncheon tables began to be somewhat predictable as recognizable alliances and friendships began to give structure to the group. Ping-Pong rivalries became fierce, and in the evenings various combinations of fellow families gave recitals on the piano, cello, clarinet, and violin.

Fault lines appeared as well. Christopher and Beth bickered about spending time with the twins. Helge began insisting that she needed time with Matteus, and brought him to lunch. "I don't see why I have to eat lunch with a ten-year-old," family-free fellows objected. "They wouldn't do it for us, because we wouldn't know how to ask," French and English families complained. Too lonely and homesick to last through the year, an African fellow went home to be with his wife and children.

"*Guten Nacht, mein kleines Kind.*" The German seemed somehow softer than the English. "Good night, my little child. Don't forget that tomorrow we get up early for physical therapy."

"*Mein kleines Mäuschen,* my little mouselet," Ned drowsily corrected me. "Frau Sonntag would say '*mein kleines Mäuschen.*'"

Tuesdays and Thursdays were my favorite mornings. It was light when I ran Ned's six o'clock bath, and sometimes we walked to physical therapy.

We were known in the cafeteria. The women made sure Ned's favorite rolls were available for him, and once the cashier gave him an old five-mark bill, a kind no longer being printed. "*Danke viel!* Thank you so much!" Ned enthused in his ever-more ready German.

Week after week Frau Sonntag and I shared Ned. We remained silent for the most part, but over time my perch in the anteroom became my place; she and other regulars would grin their welcome as I sat down with my paper and my cup of coffee.

After the half-hour I would go back to the *Kolleg* in the front seat of the 110 bus. I loved its mobile space in which I was neither scholar nor mother. I found its view more engaging than that of any living room. I noted the offerings in the theater, checked out the flower shop, gazed at the elaborate Wilmersdorff Rathaus, watched shopkeepers open their shops. As the bus swayed along, I would relax into Berlin. I arrived at the *Kolleg* primed for German class.

Appointments with Dr. Waldemeyer continued every week. In a Sunday evening phone call we would pick his freest afternoon, and, after school, Ned and I would wait in front of the hot drinks machine until he showed up. The waits could be anywhere from ten minutes to two hours long but I was learning to relax into the unstructured time. Ned and I would do homework, play cards or, if the weather was nice, he would play games among the trees. "See if you can hit the big one with a pinecone!" "Now try it with your *left* hand!" Familiar nurses would bustle past; Petra was always a possibility; once Karim was there with his father; and, if he happened by, Dr. Heller would always pause to check on "little Ned." Sooner or later Dr. Waldemeyer would come. He would bend Ned's arm back and forth and respond to its unrelenting stiffness according to his mood.

One bright afternoon, I looked up from my perch in front of the hot drinks machine to see him striding toward me, accompanied by a distinguished elderly man. They were in high professional mode, white jackets swishing as they walked and conversed. Dr. Waldemeyer looked appreciatively at Ned and me as he brought his visitor in past the hot drinks machine.

"Naja gut!" he said. "This is an interesting case that shows the work we do in my clinic. Come in!"

Dr. Waldemeyer was in a voluble mood, showing off his clinic to his appreciative visitor. I eagerly gathered informational crumbs as the two men reviewed Ned's case. They studied Dr. Schwalbach's earliest X rays and agreed that if they did not know what they were looking for they would not have seen the problem. "You see it here, but you have to look. I use the pictures for my classes," Dr. Waldemeyer said happily.

They discussed what might happen next. "It hurts him longer than I thought," Dr. Waldemeyer admitted. "But now it does not hurt so much, so physical therapy works very hard. If it does not get better in physical therapy, we do the surgery again. When there is no infection I believe that surgery can fix this problem. That is the way in this clinic."

The surgeon turned to Ned, who had waked up at this last statement. "Don't worry. You go back to America. But not yet! Now you must move your arm. You must move it and move it and move it. Then, it gets better and you do not have any more surgery."

Ned nodded and turned to me. "Can we go, Mom?" he asked.

Dr. Waldemeyer grinned at me. "I see you next week."

I smiled back, satisfied as I hadn't been in months. Finally I had answers to the questions Ned's mother was unable to ask. I had an assessment of Dr. Schwalbach's performance; I knew where Dr. Waldemeyer and his clinic stood on a spectrum of surgical aggressiveness; I had an acknowledgment of the crucial importance of the catheter infection; I had a sense of what the long-term options in Ned's case might be. I've never been more grateful than I was for the impeccably good manners that led the two Germans to carry on their conversation in English.

At the beginning of December the rector's recognition that it might require as much as a month to deal with Ned's problems had been magnanimous. But it was the middle of February, more than two months later, when the child finally emerged from the hospital, weak, depressed and in need of constant attention. By April, when I began to be ready to do more than the required minimum, Ned's demands had gone on far beyond the limits of reasonable expectation and good taste. The hothouse flowers exploded week after week from their enormous vases. The hierarchical structure of academic importance remained clear, and I was nowhere.

One lunch period I commiserated with a fellow who had broken his ankle and spent two months struggling through an operation and hospitalization. I was surprised to learn that he had been offered an additional three months to make up for the lost time. Emboldened, I made inquiries. "But, Joan," I was firmly told, "it is not the same. Holgar had a terrible accident. His ankle was very badly broken. He was more than four weeks in hospital. He had no choice."

At another lunch an American fellow pushed me to sue: Dr. Schwal-bach, Professor Mahler, Dr. Waldemeyer, someone, anyone who could be deemed responsible for what had transpired. The idea sparked a long and sophisticated discussion of the German and American legal systems, notions of responsibility, and of guilt. It was all very interesting as a set of intellectual issues, but completely irrelevant for me. I could not see how taking Ned, his arm, and his doctors into a courtroom would help me move beyond my confusions. Whatever a judge might have said, my issue was neither blame nor restitution.

It was not hard to find other interpretations among my colleagues. Intellectually the *Wissenschaftskolleg* was locked in a battle between humanists and biologists about the adequacy of biological categories for sociological understanding. When I excused myself early from a discussion that was running through the time I had to make dinner for Ned, an older fellow followed me out reassuringly. "You see? You are a mother. That is a biological category!" I didn't bother to ask what in our biology required scheduling meetings through Ned's dinner time.

The humanist interpretation of my experience was no less dismissive. "Don't worry about your work," I was told. "You have had a very rich year. You have learned a lot. You have become wise. When we men grow old we will envy you your wisdom." In the world of the *Wissenschaftskolleg*, my experience was at once absolute and illegitimate. It was consigned to the peripheral and irrational realms of biological motherhood and the wisdom of the aged.

I saw the doctors in the Otto-Hoffen-Heim, and my colleagues in the *Wissenschaftskolleg*, defending the measured calm of their worlds by creating boundaries between their public and their private, touting the public as real and dismissing the private as irrelevant detail. As I faced the ruins of my attempt to do the same I saw again how unreal but functional the whole approach is. I had often profited from it in my life and my thinking, but now it was a struggle to do either. I found it very hard to deal with my colleagues. Their clarity about our shared understanding was false, and I avoided them whenever possible.

Early morning jogs around the Grunewald See replaced my frigid walks to the Otto-Hoffen-Heim. I enjoyed watching people: the woman who always ran with her towel so she could dry off after her midrun skinny-dip, the palsied old man who made the circuit every day, the variety of dogowners with their assorted pets. One morning I encountered a wild boar with at least eight *Frischlingen,* babies; her small eyes gazed malevolently at me from her triangular face as her offspring scampered across the path about fifty feet away. At breakfast I regaled the sleepy-eyed at the *Kolleg* with my tale. "You're lucky that nothing else happened, Joan! They are really dangerous!" I had no doubt that my colleaugues were right, but I found I was more energized than frightened by my encounter. I easily understood the sow's protective ferocity.

In my office I was at work again. I had to prepare for my seminar. At the Dibner I had considered De Morgan's work in probability; at the *Wissenschaftskolleg* I followed him into logic.

The route lay through his classroom. "I have never had time for more than naturally arises out of my occupations," De Morgan once explained to Hamilton. "So that unless a question begins in something relative to teaching it does not fix my attention." At first this may seem a limited position, but for De Morgan it was not. He saw the study of mathematics to be "instrumental in furnishing the mind with new ideas, and calling into exercise some of the powers which most peculiarly distinguish man from the brute creation," and he approached his classes as the first step along a path that opened into all that was most nobly human.

Thinking logically was an essential part of this mind-expanding program. A former student affectionately described "the bland 'hush!' . . . the almost grotesque surprise he would feign when a man betrayed that, instead of the classification by logical principles, he was thinking of the old unmeaning classification by rule. . . ." The effect of his manner was "exceedingly humorous," but the point was also clear: When in De Morgan's presence the proper way to think was logically.

When he took this stand initially, De Morgan took logic to mean Aristotelian logic, in which the essential form of a valid argument is the syllogism: "All men are mortal, Socrates is a man, Therefore Socrates is mortal." Since this was the form of reasonable thought and since mathematics was a preeminently reasonable subject, De Morgan assumed, as did virtually everyone around him, that mathematical argument was logical. The only problem was that it was not always clear how to cast proofs into logical form; even the proofs of Euclid's *Elements* were not given in Aristotelian syllogisms. At first that didn't bother De Morgan, though. He saw it as a mere technicality and was quite clear that if anyone wanted to take the trouble they could make Euclid's proofs syllogistic.

However, over the course of years of trying to teach and explain mathematics logically, De Morgan began to doubt this assumption. He found it ever more difficult to interpret even the most common mathematical arguments in syllogistic form, and the closer he looked the worse the situation became. By the time he published *Formal Logic,* in 1847, De Morgan had begun to tinker with Aristotle's syllogisms in an effort to make them adequate to the demands of mathematical argument. The book was just the first step in a logical odyssey that was to engage him for the rest of his life.

In *Formal Logic,* De Morgan defined his subject as "the branch of inquiry (be it called science or art), in which the act of the mind in reasoning is considered, particularly with reference to the connection of thought and language." He defined his own interests more generally as "the examination of some of the manifestations of thinking power in their relation to the language in which they are expressed." It was a remarkably broad definition: For De Morgan logic, properly understood and developed, would describe and prescribe the way rational people actually think. "Logic is to consider the whole form of thought: *your* logic either contains the form of this thought or it does not. If it contains the form of this thought, shew it: if not, introduce it."

De Morgan's formulation of his logical challenge in terms of thought and language led him immediately into his element; a discussion of words and their meanings. In the second chapter of his *Formal Logic* his writing flows at its voluble best. "A name ought to be like a boundary, which clearly and undeniably either shuts in, or shuts out, every idea that can be suggested. It is the imperfection of our minds, our language and our knowledge of external things, that this clear and undeniable inclusion or exclusion is seldom attainable, except as to ideas which are *well within the boundary*: at and near the boundary itself all is vague." He moved seamlessly to an analogy with colors: "To the eye, green passes into blue by imperceptible gradations: our senses will suggest no place on which all agree, at which one is to end and the other to begin." From here he moved a triumphant paean to progress: "The advance of knowledge has a tendency to supply means of precise definition. . . . Wollaston and Fraunhofer [contemporary scientists] have discovered the black lines which always exist in the spectrum of solar colours given by a glass prism, in the same relative places." For De Morgan these lines marked "definite places in the spectrum, by the help of which the place of any shade of colour therein existing may be ascertained, and the means of definition given." De Morgan found this whole scenario of increasing precision to be wonderful: "It is quite within the possibilities of the application of science to the arts that the time should come when the spectrum, and the lines in it, will be used for matching colours in every linen-draper's shop," he offered in a cheery little footnote.

It was fun to read De Morgan when he was in expansive mode, but I was not sure I shared his enthusiasm for a future of absolute spectral and linguistic precision. When it comes to cloth, I rather like choosing colors with my imprecise eyes, and as for words, I was living in the shelter of their ambiguities. I was not about to trust De Morgan or anyone else to fix the meanings of *behindert* and *niederlage* for me.

But De Morgan's book soon moved from words to arguments. There, his analysis of the complex problems of convincing and being convinced was rooted in a strictly hierarchical view of the human mind and understanding. At the top was *"certainty"* which he defined as the "absolute and inassailable feeling" with which we recognize "our own existence, and that of two and two amounting to four." Below this soaring peak were "lower grades of knowledge, which we usually call *degrees of belief,* but they are really *degrees of knowledge."*

From De Morgan's point of view, beliefs could be ranged in a series from the least to the most certain, but the distinction between the most highly attested belief and perfect certainty was a difference in kind. In his *Formal Logic* he illustrated it with an example I had seen before:

> We have the lesser conviction that the pebbles at the pole fall to the ground when they are let go: we are very sure of this, without asserting that it cannot be otherwise: we see no impossibility in those pebbles being such as always to remain in air wherever they are placed. But that seven and three are not other than five and five is a matter which we are prepared to affirm as positively of the pebbles at the North Pole as of our own fingers, both that it is so, and that it *must* be so.

In De Morgan's world, certainty was absolute and unique, but there are many degrees of uncertainty.

Much of De Morgan's early logical effort was directed toward bringing mathematical order to the spectrum of uncertainty. Based on the identity of meaning between the phrases "it is more probable than improbable" and "I believe that it will happen more than I believe it will not happen," De Morgan moved to define probability theory so that it would meet his needs: "Probability then, refers to and implies belief, more or less, and belief is but another name for imperfect knowledge, or it may be, expresses the mind in a state of imperfect knowledge."

The definition leapt at me from the page and drove me from my office. I went across the street to the *Oxford English Dictionary* in the *Kolleg*'s library to confirm what Grandmama once carefully explained to me: The word *belief* comes to us from the same root as the German word *beliebt*, beloved. "Believe: To have confidence or faith in (a person) and consequently to rely upon, trust." I was relieved to find the meaning still there, still the first definition, because in this sense of the word, belief was what sustained my every day. I believed in Ned. I had believed in Dr. Lyman, in Dr. Jennings, and in Dr. Waldemeyer. I had not known what would be the outcome of Ned's operations; I now did not know whether he would ever again button his own shirt. But I believed in Ned, and I believed in his doctors. My belief in them was not a statement of imperfect knowledge.

At first De Morgan had nodded, albeit feebly, to the distinction between Grandmama's and my personal understanding of the word *belief* and his epistemological one: What "we usually call *degrees of belief* . . . are really *degrees of knowledge*," he admitted. But then he let the distinction go, and gaily launched into his analysis of degrees of belief. Each time he quantified *belief* in this way, the word lost some of its magic, until finally, utterly exhausted, it lay pinned to his page like a fading butterfly.

As I returned to my office and contemplated *belief*'s newly truncated meaning, I realized I'd seen this process before. I'd seen the word *relativity* moved from a position of personal power to one of human weakness. I'd been watching the word *moral* switch between a similar position of power—as in Sophia's judgement that Ellis possessed "an almost perfect moral character"—and the weakness of Augustus's throwaway "moral probabilities." All of these words, and many more besides, had fallen victim to a larger drive to find mathematical certainties in an uncertain world.

The consequences were dramatic. De Morgan was so intent on his search for logical certainty that his own daughter's sparkling arctic world of flying birds and kissing Eskimos was frozen into cold and rigid absolutes. I understood the justification for his efforts, the reasons for his attempt to find a rational world in which people could communicate across religious differences. It was a noble vision, one that had always overcome my doubts and struggles in the past. But in Berlin I saw that the price was just too high. Even if he were to succeed in his logical program, I could not rejoice in the world that he was constructing.

The closest De Morgan came to understanding the issue that divided us was in the context of the four-color problem. The connection was tenuous at best, a map is not a person, but in this context I could watch him struggle to understand a situation in which he found himself completely convinced about something that he could not rationally substantiate. When he first asked Hamilton whether four colors would be enough to distinguish all countries on any map, he noted: "It is tricky work, and I am not sure of all convolutions." But only a couple of sentences later, he mused: "The more I think of it the more evident it seems." By the time he sent the problem to Whewell in December of the following year, De Morgan was secure enough in his conviction that he could describe its development. He found the four-color idea "at first incredible—then certainly true—then axiomatic—for I cannot make it depend on anything I see more clearly."

I have never had any trouble admitting the absolute truth of the four-color problem: A few tries have always been enough to render it obvious, just as De Morgan said they would. But I did have trouble with the narrow compass of interpretation he allowed for understanding his and my conviction. It troubled De Morgan too, and he reached for assurance with his letters. Lacking a proof, he searched for consensus, urging friends to try it for themselves and even to test other people: "But you must speak doubtingly yourself—as if it were not settled in your own mind."

But the depth of his unsubstantiated conviction about truth of the four-color problem was not strong enough to make De Morgan rethink his bifurcated world of absolute certainty and imperfect belief. Ultimately, he just neutralized the problem by sticking it, however awkwardly, into the world of simple absolutes. Subsequent generations refused to accept that the four-color conjecture was axiomatic, but its ambivalent status was not enough to make them modify their understanding of the nature and bases of certainty, either. The millions of hours of labor that have been expended on efforts to prove the four-color problem are a monument to the modern determination to save the world of absolute truths that De Morgan found so compelling.

Sticking to the nineteenth century, I was relieved to find that many of De Morgan's contemporaries found his approach as claustrophobic as I did. From the moment he published *Formal Logic* in 1847 he was embroiled in ferocious controversies. Much of the heat was generated by a fight with a Scottish philosopher, William Hamilton (no relation of De Morgan's Irish correspondent), who, with no clear justification but egotistical ill humor, accused De Morgan of plagiarism. It was a stupid argument that spluttered for decades and unfortunately tended to mask the substantive issues that lay behind objections to De Morgan's logic.

There were real objections, however. Two years after *Formal Logic* was published, I found Ellis writing indignantly against probabilistic attempts to mathematically order degrees of belief: *"Avec les chiffres on peut tout demontrer* [With numbers one can demonstrate anything] ought to be the motto of most of the philosophical applications of the theory of probabilities. . . . To attempt to constitute it into the philosophy of science is, in effect to destroy the philosophy of science altogether."

Ellis wrote his remarks in a private letter, but Henry Longueville Mansel, an Oxford theologian, blasted De Morgan's logical program in a review published in 1851. The article quickly devolves into a swirl of subtle arguments drawn from Kant, Hegel, and many more besides. But behind all of his rhetoric, Mansel was basically defending a simple position. He was insisting that De Morgan's logical approach to the world was not adequate to all of human thought.

De Morgan had always been leery of German philosophy. Just two years before Mansel's review appeared, he had admitted in a letter to Whewell: "I stop at Kant, whom I spell with a C and an apostrophe; I c'an't get through him," But De Morgan loved nothing more than a good fight about logic, and even the horrors of Kant could not hold him back from an engagement with Mansel. In his four-color-problem letter to Whewell he was laying some of the groundwork for his counterattack.

But then Alice died, and her father went silent. De Morgan slowly regained his equilibrium, though, and by the time ten years had passed he could describe himself as "routing in my book like a pig in a potato garden, who does not need much care where his snout goes, as he is sure of finding something." In a series of seminal articles beginning in 1858 he responded to Mansel and further developed his logic. Time and experience did not temper De Morgan's logical imperialism any more than the four-color problem had, however. In his later logical writings he was, if anything, more committed than ever to the pursuit of his universalizing program.

Day after day in Berlin I disciplined myself to read the Mansel–De Morgan debate, but I found little that was helpful to me in either side of the tangle of convoluted argument and technical detail. My issue leapt out at me one morning as I was reading De Morgan's correspondence with his pen-pal and fellow logician, George Boole. In 1862, Boole who lived in Ireland, complained about his intellectual isolation. "There is absolutely no person in this country except my wife with whom I ever speak on subjects like this," he wrote as he thanked De Morgan for sending a paper. From his study in the middle of London,

De Morgan responded: "I have not *one* person to whom I can speak on logic. . . ."

My mind flew to the frontispiece of my copy of De Morgan's *Formal Logic*. It was a black-and-white reproduction of a pastel portrait Sophia drew just before she and Augustus were married. It was clearly a work of love that took Augustus straight on, his right eye staring blindly out from behind his thick glasses. I contemplated it and thought of a letter that Sophia had included in her *Memoir*.

To J. S. Mill, Esq., MP

91 Adelaide Rd, August 2, 1867

My Dear Sir, —

As touching your proposal to me to join the committee of the National Society for Women's Suffrage, I cannot accede. . . . Your Society, as its title is worded, contemplates a full female suffrage—*e.g.* a vote for a man and another for his wife. Supposing me willing to join a political agitation, I should hardly be ready for such a one as this. I should think better of two votes given to the couple jointly—*i.e.* the two to agree upon the two. I almost thought this was the meaning of the phrase 'compound house-holder' when I first heard people mention it.

Even the ever-loving and supportive Sophia was unable to let this letter go by without response. In one of the very few modifying footnotes of the *Memoir* she commented: "I cannot help thinking my husband wrote this for the sake of playing on the expression 'compound householder,' as he can scarcely have missed seeing that the result of one vote to each of two people has the exact effect of two votes to both, if they agree, except only in the case of one of the two not voting at all."

The whole interchange revealed to me a Sophia who was at once highly intelligent, crisply alert, and remarkably nonjudgmental. What little I could glean of her from all that I had read, supported my view that she was highly engaged in making meaningful sense of her world. No wonder I could make so little sense of my experience in Augustus's terms! He had not included his wife in his construction of the rational.

5/16/96

Dear Rick,

Yesterday was a good day—I wrote a bit! which distracted me to such an extent that I was late to lunch. When I got there, though, there was Jonathon Foley. It was such a rush of excitement to see someone from home. Gave me a sense of what it might be like to actually get there. Invited him to dinner and then had to shop, realizing in the "nick of time" that *Himmelfahrt* [Ascension] means all would be closed today. So I laid up provisions—too many to carry comfortably—which Ned and Sean rowed back in the boat. Great joy somewhere along the line because Sean managed to fall in. Once back a flurry to warm Sean up and get the two off to baseball. Pleasant supper with Jonathon, Brady was out late for dinner with "Sue." She has been a name since the fall; how does she fit in with Julie, Marina, and Rosemary? I can't follow the social life of a 16-year-old. Little boys back and to bed and today is *Himmelfahrt*. Somewhere in the bustle, my material from Cambridge arrived which is exciting though it may be hard to find a way to read it today. Sigh! I wish the schools would just keep them for a bit.

5/16/96

Dear Joan,

Just got back from walking Bil and decided to check in prior to leaving for work. Glad Brady has a social life although somewhat serial in nature. Sorry Ned has to be free to observe *Himmelfahrt,* perhaps he ought to be in church somewhere to do this right. I'm off to confront work with a lighter heart having heard from you.

The desultory pace of baseball held no charms for me that spring; I had had my fill of empty time in the Otto-Hoffen-Heim. But Ned was a pitcher in Berlin's tiny little league. Every Saturday morning he would take off early, with his bat and his glove, a grin and a wave. "I struck someone out!" "I pitched a no-hitter!" As the spring progressed I could almost see the wing feathers of his resilient self sprouting from his cap.

Week after week Ned pressed me to watch him pitch, until finally one gray June morning I took my place in the rickety bleachers alongside a sprinkling of other parents. Ned's team was batting and the game was somewhat tortuous; the pitching was spotty and many walked. Finally, though, there was enough action to change sides. Ned cheerily donned his mitt and went out to pitch. His teammates chattered their support and he beamed.

Then he faced the batter. You could see him focus, his strong, athletic body poised for the windup. Dr. Jennings's scar was a barely perceptible line in the hair below his cap. He drew the ball toward his chin with both hands, his stiff elbow forcing him to stop short of the full tuck. Then he unwound and hurled the ball toward the plate. "Ball one!" the demanding umpire called.

The catcher threw the ball back to Ned. Again he wound up and pitched.

"Strike one!" the umpire called.

"Timothy, Ned is pitching. You better swing," the other team's coach called.

Ned wound and pitched again: "Strike two!"

The woman next to me in the bleachers said to her husband "That kid can pitch!"

"Strike three!" the umpire called.

Ned leaned slightly to the left in order to snag the ball the catcher had thrown. He tossed it from glove to hand and back again; he meditatively kicked the earth on the mound.

I was suddenly sad that Dr. Waldemeyer could not see him in this role. Had he been there the German might have been at a loss to understand this quintessentially American game, and the doctor unable to see how UN-*behindert* this child was. But I wanted the rest of him to see what I could see as I watched Ned calmly and firmly eyeing the next batter: Whatever had happened during the long Berlin winter the child had emerged whole.

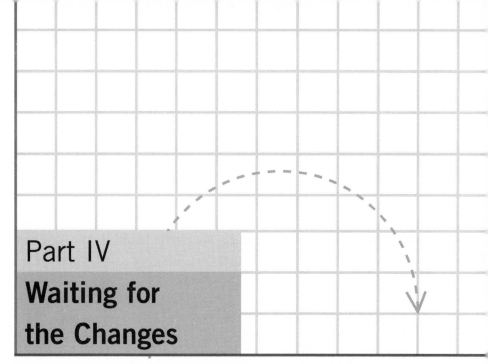

Part IV
Waiting for the Changes

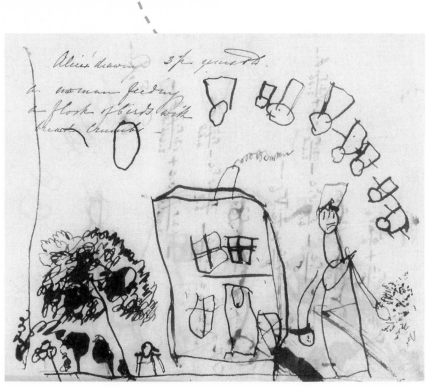

"Alice's drawing. 3½ years old. A woman feeding a flock of birds with bread crumbs." De Morgan Foundation Archive, De Morgan Foundation, London.

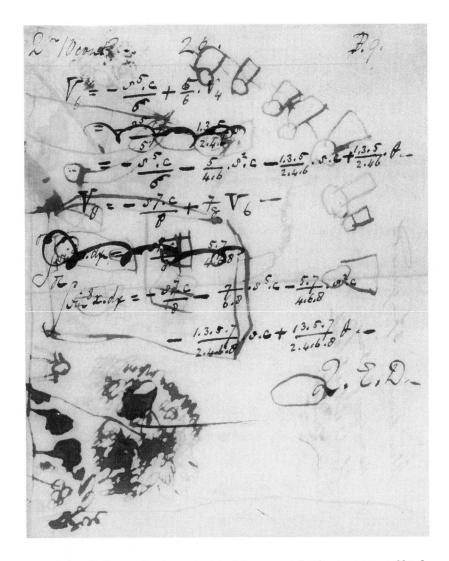

Autograph calculations by Augustus De Morgan, with Alice's picture of birds bleeding through from the other side. De Morgan Foundation Archive, De Morgan Foundation, London.

America (*Amerika*)

Through most of the month of June, when Berlin's spring should have been ripening into summer, it poured. A flood turned the Kurfürstendamm into a river. Manhole covers burst up on Koenigsallee. The swans were flooded off of their island, and Dr. Geisler's MRI machine was ruined by the water. Ned's June pictures for Dr. Jennings were among the first to be taken on a brand new machine.

One lowering Tuesday in June, I gave my seminar in the formal space of the *Wissenschaftskolleg* seminar room. The fellows sat in force around the table; those from the Max Planck Institute sat in the back rows. Families, both mine and De Morgan's, were decorously absent. But I was acutely aware of them. Even as I spoke of logic, I recognized that its definition created by default a separate sphere to house all the contradictory realities that families represented. But even as I did what was expected I realized that I was never again going to be able blithely to follow De Morgan or my colleagues without noticing what their thinking implied for their wives and for me.

There were no significant developments on the medical front. Physical therapy continued, but Ned's motion did not improve particularly. Opinions about what he might do in the future varied considerably. Dr. Waldemeyer said, "He could always have the operation again, Mrs. Richards. Now he knows what it means to move with pain. Maybe when he is sixteen or eighteen, he decides he wants to try to move it more." Frau Sonntag contemplated the scars on his arm in dismay and said fiercely. "*Nie wieder,* never again, *Frau Richards! Nie wieder!*" I didn't have to choose between them, though. All agreed that we had done what we could for now and that future decisions could wait until Ned was old enough to make them for himself.

For the moment all Ned wanted was to go home. He began to count down. "Only thirteen more days of school!" "Only six more times in physical therapy!" "Only one more appointment with Dr. Waldemeyer!"

❖ ❖ ❖

"So, Ned. You come back to Germany sometimes? You come back to see me sometimes?"

I nudged Ned to attention. He focused enough to answer. "No, I don't think so."

Rebuffed, the doctor looked at me. Eight months of caring accommodation lay between us—eight months of steadfast presence: returned phone calls, appointments on days off.

"Of *course* we'll come back to Berlin sometime. And of course we'll come to see you," I offered. It was the best I could come up with in the terms allowed between mother and doctor, but it was pretty feeble.

On his side, Ned's surgeon could do no better. "Keep moving your arm, Ned. You can always lean on it like this." He repeated the familiar demonstration against the wall.

"OK," Ned said.

Petra gave Ned a book, we took pictures of him playing with Frau Sonntag, there were hugs, kisses, and tears all around—all except for Ned, who was in no mood for tears.

"Tomorrow, Mom!"

The next morning Brady helped me get Ned and his luggage to the airport where I turned my son over to the stewardess. "*Tchuss,* bro! Good-bye, Mom! See you in America!" Schnell's eyes gleamed from under his arm and Racky looked back from his knapsack as Ned followed the young woman to the plane and to his father.

Brady didn't leave for another week but he was so busy with his friends that I virtually never saw him. For a month my family telescoped into daily e-mail messages.

7/5/96

Dear Joan,

It's 5 pm and already I've piled up quite a day with Ned. He began the day by appearing at my bedside at 5 am asking what time it was, saying that he didn't believe what the clock in his room was telling him (this may have to do with the issue of being able to read clock faces.) Anyway, that was that. I dozed a little and got up. We spent time unpacking and putting things away, which led to laundry, dishes, and other domestic odds and ends. Then on to Ann & Hope where we did a pretty good shopping for camp (oh yes, stopping first at the shoe store where we got sneakers and Tevas). We also got a watch with the classic face because Ned said he needed the discipline to make him learn how to tell time that way.

Then somewhat to my surprise we went to Chili's for lunch, complete with Awesome Blossom. Then home to unload shopping bags, call James about the gerbils, get the MRIs and X rays and set off for Dr. Lyman. He was nice, as was Janet. Dr. Lyman confessed he felt somewhat bad sending Ned off to camp, but said he was going to anyway but Ned should take every opportunity to exercise the elbow and not be a lazy lout. He was most impressed at how abruptly the extension and flexion ends—wham! that's it! We see a physical therapist this Wednesday and an orthopedic pediatrician after camp.

Then we were off to Rainbow bikes, where we ordered Ned a bike that should be ready by the end of camp. Then to the grocery store: Jerry [our next-door neighbor] is coming for dinner and we want to barbecue. And on to home.

Then over to James's house to pick up the gerbils, and back again. I've put some coffee on in the hopes it may revive me. My feet hurt and I want to lie down, but Ned is out weed-whacking in the back yard. If I can only get him to clean up! Hope all is well and will write tomorrow if I have the strength.
Love, Rick

7/10/96

Dear Joan,

We saw the physical therapist today, who is worried about Ned and camp. She wonders whether he should go at all. Wherever he is, though, she thinks he should keep up physical therapy at least once a day. What do you think?
Love, Rick

7/10/96

Dear Rick,

I don't care if his arm falls off. Ned has to go to camp. I'll call Dr. Lyman if you like. . . . Love, Joan

7/15/96

Dear Joan,

Yesterday was sunny around here with fog moving in during the evening. With Ned at camp I am focusing on Brady. He's a walking commentary on the differences between German and American culture. We went out to dinner last night. He gave me a long dissertation on "bland," "flavor," and "taste," semimystical qualities that seem to me to have to do with the intensity of the experience. Anyway, coffee has taste and tea has flavor—just remember that. Also, he had just showered and had his bangs combed straightforward so they came down to his nose. Looking at his eyes through this fringe was very disconcerting, so I demanded he part them. He did so and we had a long talk about looking into people's eyes. He is without doubt deep into the art of conversation. I'm going to have to get with it!

I spent most of the final month of my fellowship alone in Berlin. The weekly seminars continued unabated: global warming, medieval mysticism, clonal plants. Lunches and dinners went on as well. Then, in mid-July, there was a farewell party, followed by the slow drifting-away of the fellows.

When not formally engaged I was in my office. With my seminar done, I was free of De Morgan, of logic, of mathematics. People suggested that, as an alternative, I write a comparative study of the American and German health systems, but I was in no mood to confine my thinking to the analytic space carved out by an academic project; to make a clear point, defend a position, establish a truth. I had a story to tell, and I spent hours in my office writing it.

When I'd had enough of reminiscences, I searched for Alice. I knew it was a fool's errand; almost one hundred fifty years of historical erasure stood between De Morgan's daughter and me. But I kept looking. I wanted desperately to find her.

My search was very frustrating. Sophia noted, at the end of her *Memoir*, that her husband "never liked making known what nearly concerned his family," and she was right. I scoured his letters but in vain. De Morgan was always willing to ask about and respond to his friends' families, but about his own he was silent. Hamilton, in particular, cheerfully shared little tidbits. "This is my little daughter's twelfth birthday. . . . The red ink is a birthday present *from her*, which I found on my pillow, in a parcel with pens, &c., when I awoke pretty early this morning; *that* is always *her* notion of *her* birthday, that *she* is to make the presents." De Morgan responded by sending puzzles, but no corresponding sketches of Alice or others of his children.

The closest I could come was a parenthetical reference: "Citation leads to queer results sometimes. At the Lady's College in Bedford-square (where my daughter goes) the teacher of mathematics quoted me about logarithms in his class; and my daughter heard one of the girls saying 'Oh, I wish Mr. De Morgan had never invented those logarithms.'" Alice would have been about fourteen at the time. I saw her in some kind of Victorian uniform, a student at a school for girls. I was glad she was being educated, and the scene gave me a glimpse of her power over her father. I saw that it was because of Alice that Augustus came to modify his "manly views of women," and to cooperate with Sophia's work on behalf of female education.

It was something, but very small. I wanted more. It was in a biography of Alice's brother that I had found Sophia's nursery diary quoted at such length; I called archivists all over England in quest of the original, but to no avail. Then one chilly June afternoon I realized that a letter from Hamilton contained a possibility.

WRH to ADM, December 17, 1853

Your note of the 15th ought perhaps to have reached me yesterday instead of this morning; and, if so, I should sooner have expressed my sympathy in your parental anxiety for your daughter, at an interesting time of her life, and important crisis of her health. You know how apt I am to talk, at least to *you* (for I am somewhat more guarded with people in general), about my *own* daughter. . . . I have been showing *my* child Helen (what is *your* daughter's name?), at her own wish, ever so many astronomical things to-day—not that she understands them all.

What is your daughter's name? It was Alice! Finally aware that she was ill, had De Morgan worked through his anxieties by writing about her in the week before she died? If so, the editor of my volume of letters, who did not include De Morgan's letter in his edition, had erased her as effectively as everyone else had. I began writing to friends who had worked in the Hamilton archives to try to spark memories of a letter about Alice.

When I'd had enough of my office, I wandered about Berlin. It was lonely without the boys and I felt adrift without the Otto-Hoffen-Heim as a point of reference. In defense I attached myself shamelessly to anyone who would accept my company. I went on a boat trip through the Wannsee and the rivers I'd not been able to skate. I visited Sans Souci, the eighteenth-century jewel that was a palace of Sophia Charlotte's grandson, Friedrich II. I toured the site of the Wannsee Conference, where Hitler's henchmen decided that genocide was the "final solution" to the "Jewish question." The Philharmonie was on summer vacation but I went out to dinner, to a jazz club, to movies, to plays.

One hot afternoon I bicycled to a farther, larger *See* than the one I was used to, with an American fellow's wife. It was hot and we were sticky. Suddenly, at the same moment, it struck her that we were not in Puritan America, me that we were not in Victorian England. Grinning wickedly we took off all of our clothes and went skinny-dipping. The Berliners strolling by paid no attention at all.

And so, time passed pleasantly but slowly; by the end of the month I was ready to go. On Thursday, July 30, I flew away from Berlin. By this time Brady had gone off to be with my mother for the summer and Ned was still at camp. I arrived for a week alone with Rick.

During the days I tried to get used to being in a place where Berlin and my life in it were simply an exotic irrelevance. "Joan! Is that you? How was Berlin? I bet you're glad to be back!" "Joan! Two years' leave, you lucky dog! How's your book?" I really had no answers to these questions; to avoid them I searched out the peace of the garden.

In the evenings, when Rick got back from work, he and I were together. We went to a grocery store, so huge to my German-accustomed eyes that I could barely move. But Rick was used to picking up little bits here and there to make small dinners; he took charge of the shopping. Sometimes we went out to dinner, sometimes we went to movies. Mostly we were at home. We had a lot of catching up to do, stories to tell, fences to mend. We had been far apart for a very long time.

At the end of the week we went together to pick up Ned. Somehow the time away had made his elbow seem less strange and restricted. We were all getting used to the situation. Or were we? In the next day or two I kept watching Ned. I watched him un-self-consciously reach for the breadbasket at dinner. I noticed him reading in bed, his head propped on his left hand. Could he do those things before? I looked forward eagerly to his appointment with the physical therapist. I was curious to know his angles.

The woman greeted us with the warm friendliness I have come to associate with the profession. She eyed Ned's elbow and said, "Looks good. Let's warm it up a bit and see what we've got." She set Ned up to pedal a stationary arm bicycle, two and a half minutes in one direction, two and a half in the other. Then she laid him on the table and measured his angles. "Zero to minus 17 degrees to 127," she said. The terminology was strange but the message clear. Four happy weeks of freedom had done what all of our focused efforts had been unable to accomplish. Finally, at home again, Ned could easily eat an apple, button a shirt, or tie a tie.

"*Frau Sonntag* HAT *den elbogen* BEWEGT. Frau Sonntag moved the elbow." Transitive verb, action on an object. "*Ned* HAT *den elbogen* BEWEGT. Ned moved the elbow." Transitive verb, action on an object. "*Der elbogen* HAT BEWOGEN. The elbow moved." Intransitive verb, action contained by the object. I sent pictures to Petra and Frau Sonntag. I suspected they could understand it all more easily than I.

✻ ✻ ✻

In the meantime, Brady returned from my mother's, and both boys started school. I did as well. "Good morning. I am Professor Richards from the history department and this is History 118, The Rise of the Scientific Worldview. . . ."

In the evenings we came from our far-flung days to be again a family foursome in our little dining room. Rick's jokes were as bad as ever.

"What did the duck say when he walked out of the bar? . . . You give up? . . . 'Just put it on my bill.'"

"Mom! Where did you find him?" Brady wailed.

Ned was unperturbed. "Dad, come on! I haven't done my pull-up for today."

After supper Rick took Ned to work his arm on the bars at the Hope High School Field. Brady did the dishes and then retired to his room.

"Have you written to colleges asking for applications, Brady?"

"Don't worry, Mom. I know what I'm doing."

"Hey, Mom!" Ned burst in breathless. "I went all the way across on the monkey bars!" Rick brought up the rear, grinning with pride. The telephone rang. "Brady there?"

Ned sat on Dr. Gasparian's examining table while the neurologist flipped through the telephone book of scribbly EEG lines. "Looks good!" he said. "We'll keep him on Tegretol for another year."

Ned roused himself from his doze. "If I'm fine, why do I have to take Tegretol?" But Dr. Gasparian still was not one to answer questions: "You don't want another seizure, do you?"

Seeing Dr. Jennings was rather like seeing the unmasked Wizard of Oz. We reached him on our first try, and without the surgery hanging over us, he was not terrifying. He was suitably impressed by the pictures Dr. Geisler had sent and agreed there were no problems.

"Did you learn to speak German in Germany, Edward?"

"*Ja,*" Ned said with a yawn.

"I understand that Ned has to see an orthopedic surgeon, Dr. Lyman, but we're both rather skittish. No one is going to operate on him in the foreseeable future."

"I hear you! You may have to wait, but make an appointment with Dr. Pagel. Ned will like him. He's very good with kids."

Brady was in school. Ned was in school. Rick was at work. I was in my office. A student knocked and opened my door.

"Professor Richards? I'm Amanda Schwarz. I'm a student in History 118 and I have a question about Newton and Leibniz."

"OK."

"They argued about space, right? Newton thought things were true but Leibniz said that everything is just relative. Right?"

I was engulfed in a wave of response: "*Sei tapfer!*" "*There is nothing wrong!*" "*I'll have grounds more relative than this.*" "*Ned has to begin to live again.*" "*What if I send the file?*" "*When many things are seen together one perceives that order of things among themselves.*" "*I think the situation is completely normal.*" "Hush!" De Morgan said to my unquiet mind.

"Well, let's look at the texts," I said. "Where are you confused?"

Amanda and I went over the passages that were troubling her just as we would have before my sabbatical, and Amanda left satisfied.

Alone at my desk I was not satisfied. Newton and Leibniz were all entwined with Berlin and Ned and his doctors. I could not address them from my Providence office.

At the end of October, Ned and I went to see Dr. Pagel. The man stood at least six feet, two inches, and gave the impression he had played intermural football in college. "Hello Sport! So, you're the kid with all the German operation reports! How's your arm now? . . . Wow! Look at that! A double capsulotomy! Magnificent! I'd have to go for a six-week course in Switzerland to learn how to do that. Let's see you move it." Ned moved his arm up and down with the fluid motion I was becoming accustomed to. "Let's see the angles . . . extension to 15 degrees . . . flexion to 135 degrees."

"One hundred thirty-five degrees?" Had Ned gained nine degrees since he'd come home from camp?

"Yup!" Dr. Pagel said, and showed me on his goniometer. I noted the date and wrote the numbers on the angle-measure page of the yellow notebook.

Dr. Pagel moved Ned's arm up and down, shaking his head in amazement. "Incredible!" he said. "You're lucky you were in Germany. That guy really knew what he was doing."

At the house, Rick's garden lay tangled in the fullness of the fall. Ripening tomatoes bent their branches to the ground and some kind of volunteer squash was entwined over all. Brady's jacket hung from the back fence; he must have decided it was not going to rain as he mounted his bicycle for school. Ned was also in school, perhaps with his head propped on his left hand.

October 26, 1996

Dear Dr. Waldemeyer,

When you operated on Ned in January, you projected that he would lose about 10 degrees of motion on each side of the 0-10-140 movement you got under anesthetic. Enclosed is a picture of Ned flexing his elbow at the end of four weeks at camp. You can't tell the exact measurements but I think you can see how good it is. A month ago the physical therapist rejected him because he is fully functional. This morning Dr. Pagel measured his angles and found them to be 0-15-135. CONGRATULATIONS!

    Joan L. Richards

I took the little yellow notebook out of the zippered compartment of my purse where I had carried it for two years. As I flipped through its pages brimming with instructions, telephone numbers, measurements, and questions I realized how false my letter was. I wrote it because I both hoped and thought Dr. Waldemeyer would be glad to get it; it was the right letter to write. But in this form I knew that he would not get it, not really. Something much bigger had happened than an operation on a child's left elbow.

Something much bigger had happened, but I could neither understand nor deal with it. "Joan," I told myself firmly, "it is not a time for tears nor for this book. Ned does not have any more doctors' appointments." I bound the notebook's yellow cover and its various slips together with a rubber band, and stuck it in a cubby in my desk. It was time for the story to be done.

A Quiet Business

I was resolute, but shelving the yellow notebook was a bit like bedding a child before its time. It popped up again in March for a follow-up appointment with Dr. Pagel. "Four degrees more extension!" he said heartily. "That's really amazing!" It came out again for a May appointment with Dr. Gasparian, who broke through his gloom enough to pronounce Ned "much better" and take him off Tegretol. It came out yet again for an early June appointment with Dr. Jennings, who said that Ned's recovery was "marvelous."

Gradually time dulled the immediacy of my confusion, and I got used to the pain of contemplating all the work I had not done. Still, I could not pick it up again; I could not accept what had happened; I could not come to terms with all that had been lost. In the evenings I studied German as if somehow, if I understood the language, I could understand what had happened there. In the days I taught my courses dutifully and conservatively, but my mind was like a restless child, tossing and turning and messing up the covers.

One morning in March, at least eight months after I'd begun inquiring after Alice, I received a little packet from an Irish archive. I raced to a microfilm machine.

Dec. 15, 1853

My dear Hamilton,

I have two notes to answer—one just rec.d—but must defer till a future time. I had hardly seen my mother out of danger when my eldest daughter (aged 15½) was attacked with a gradually growing fever which now places her in great danger—we are afraid of rapid decline (pulmonary) coming on immediately. A few days will settle whether the fever can be so far reduced as to give time to meet the other danger.

Yours sincerely,

A. De Morgan

7 Camdn St

Jan. 10/54

Dear Hamilton

I think, if I remember right, that I wrote you a short note, telling you how completely the illness of my eldest daughter prevented my even reading your notes—On the 23d of last month she died, in her sixteenth year, of a complication of nervous fever, inflammation of the lungs and very rapid development of tubercles, as appeared by the examination which I thought it right to have made. That she escaped the slow and melancholy process of common tubercular disorder is the consolation, such as it is, which ✳ gives on this side of the great change which we call death.

I am just beginning to recover—I will not say my spirits—but power enough to attend to things not absolutely essential.—I shall take your different notes soon—I read them hurriedly as rec.d—and have quite forgotten the contents—in fact, all my papers look as they might if I had been suddenly carried off, all round the world, and set down again at my desk.

I was overwhelmed. I don't know what I had expected but what I got was somehow more than I bargained for. A world of lost meaning rushed into and out of the unreadable blot ✳, a little square of petrified rubber band somehow left there by a careless archivist. I knew De Morgan would have been very careful about the word he chose, but I would never know what gives the consolation. *"He always dwelt on the belief that those whom God loves are the early taken, but after we lost Alice his cheerfulness diminished, and I do not think he ever laughed so heartily, or was heard whistling and singing merry snatches of songs as he used to do when all our children were with us. I cannot write of these events."*

That spring, between lectures, committee meetings, and little-league games I reread the end of Sophia's *Memoir*. It was very sad. In 1866 De Morgan quarreled with University College over a hiring decision.

When Mr. De Morgan heard that the Council intended to reject Mr. Martineau for reasons connected with religious belief, he openly declared that should the College make such a departure from the principle on which it was founded, he should feel that his connection with it was at an end. He waited with anxiety for their decision, and when the news came that the acknowledged best candidate was set aside on the ground of his

Unitarianism . . . he did not hesitate as to his own course, but at once sent in his resignation. . . .

The reading of [his] letter at the Council was (I [Sophia] was told) followed by silence for a minute or two. . . . The secretary was directed to inform the writer 'that your letter of November 10, addressed to the Chairman of the Council, was read at a session of the Council on Saturday last, and that your resignation of the Professorship of Mathematics from the close of the current session was accepted.'

Thus, after almost forty happy years devoted entirely to teaching there, De Morgan was let go from his beloved college.

The next year Augustus received another blow. Still in his twenties, his second son, George was well on his way to following in his father's mathematical footsteps, when he succumbed to tuberculosis. "I bear it well, and so does my wife," Augustus wrote to John Herschel the day after the funeral.

But Augustus did not bear it well. In the next year his "health, which had continued steadily to decline, broke down entirely. A sharp attack of congestion of the brain, the result of so much intense mental suffering, left him so prostrated that it was evident he never again would be equal to sustained effort." A feeble old man in his early sixties, Augustus began to focus his search for meaning on the words of the Bible, "reading the Greek Testament, and comparing the different versions and translations."

The image of Augustus reaching for understanding by fixing more and more exactly the meanings of the words in his Bible seemed too much to bear, but his trials were still not over.

In August, 1870, seven months before his own release, our daughter Christiana was taken [also from tuberculosis]. . . . I [Sophia] came home the day after her death to find her father so weak that he had that day fallen on the floor, and was unable to rise without help.

From this time the decline in his health was very apparent, but he did not seem to suffer, except from weakness and sleeplessness. The physical state was a complicated one, chiefly owing to nervous prostration, and traceable in the first instance to the shock of the College disappointment, and afterwards to anxiety and sorrow on our children's account. . . . During the last two days of his life . . . he seemed to recognise all those of his family whom he had lost—his three children, his mother and sister, whom he greeted, naming them in the reverse order to that in which they left this world. . . . After this he said very little, only on the last morning of his life asking me, as he had been used to do, 'if it was time to get up.' On being told that it would soon be, he seemed to be carefully dressing himself. Then he lay quite still till, just after midnight, he breathed his last.

The last years of Augustus's life hit me with an almost physical pain, but as I read I found myself thinking about Sophia as much as about her subject. Her writing about the final break with the University College her father had helped found and her husband had served so well was firm and clear. Her description of the death of her husband and their children was calm and strong. Augustus was completely broken by the collapse of his rational world, but Sophia was not. I had spent years reading about Augustus and months searching for Alice. Now I wanted to find Sophia.

I looked again at the two works Sophia had written about her family, but the *Memoir* remained inexorably about Augustus and her autobiography about other prominent people. There was another book, though, which I had never been tempted to read. Even in the period following Ned's neurosurgery my interest in the De Morgans had not been enough to draw me into the world of late nineteenth-century spiritualism: the world of walking ghosts, listening mediums, and rapt table-turners. But Sophia had been deeply involved in this world and I wanted to find her. So, one blustery April day I went to the library and checked out *From Matter to Spirit* by C. D. with a preface by A. B. Under C. D., a librarian with a neat nineteenth-century hand had carefully penned, "(Mrs. Augustus [Sophia Elizabeth] De Morgan)"; under A. B., "(Professor Augustus De Morgan)."

My first move was to leaf through the crumbling book in search of Alice. "For obvious reasons names are suppressed and initials changed," Sophia explained, but I quickly identified her daughter. "This young girl is Ellen;" a medium observed, "quite herself, so fresh, and fair and young. She is looking at me with her bright smile from behind a rose-bush; she seems to be just pushing aside the branches to let me see her face. Now I see that with the other hand she holds the hand of a noble-looking old man whom she calls [grandfather]." Another time a seer "described herself as *'seeing'* or *'being in,'* a very lovely park, in which were trees loaded with blossoms, and grass gemmed with bright flowers. Children were playing on the grass in groups, making wreaths of the flowers, and all seemed a picture of beauty and happiness. 'Among the children,' the [seer] said, 'I see some young people and some who are old, or elderly. There is Ellen and M—[Sophia's father] . . .'" I found these passages sadly insipid in comparison to the Alice I had read about before. Still, I was glad that Sophia had found a way to understand her loss that left her child unharmed, happy, and beloved by her family.

But Sophia's glimpses of Alice constitute only a very little part of her book, which runs to almost 400 pages, including notes. In the rest of it she painstakingly combined her experiences with those of others, constructed from them a complex geography of the world after death, and then mapped the progress of souls through that world.

A major part of Sophia's initial challenge was to locate her book in the public realm by establishing the scientific validity of her experiences. These scientific aspirations explain the presence of Augustus's preface; he was using his authority to defend the authenticity of her account. "I am perfectly convinced that I have both seen and heard in a manner which should make unbelief impossible, things *called* spiritual," Sophia's husband proclaimed. He was less clear in his support for his wife's interpretations of those experiences: "When it comes to what is the cause of these phenomena, I find I cannot adopt any explanation which has yet been suggested." Nonetheless, he insisted, "The spiritualists, beyond a doubt, are in the track that has led to all advancement in physical science: their opponents are the representatives of those who have striven against progress," and he devoted the rest of his almost fifty-page preface to defending the legitimacy of her effort.

Even as Augustus wrote in support of Sophia's enterprise, he proclaimed: "Both the author and myself had substantially finished before either set eyes on what the other had written." This was, I realized, an attempt on his part to assert his objectivity, but I had no trouble believing it to be true. Sophia's first chapter is entitled "Introductory—Method of Experimenting," but her approach to her subject was absolutely different from anything I had found in Augustus.

In his thinking about logic and probabilities Augustus had defined out of consideration all situations in which the actor's personal processes might be implicated in the proceedings, but people's inner states absolutely controlled the outcome of all of Sophia's experiments. If members of a party did not "preserve a really religious, earnest, and truth-loving spirit," they might well be visited by spirits who "seem to delight only in bufoonery or abuse" and play "absurd and mischievous tricks" like giving as their names "Richard Couer de Lion, Pythagoras, Byron, Cheops, and Mr. Fauntleroy." Time and time again Sophia emphasized the importance of working with people who were constructively committed to the experience.

Sophia did not just have to rely on others to cooperate in sessions with her, however. She distilled her view of the afterlife from the testimonies of a remarkably diverse group of people including servants, children, neighbors, Plato, St. Paul, Swedenbourg, and, of course, mediums. On first meeting she used little tricks to test their basic truthfulness: "I tried to test her [a newly hired servant girl] by suggesting additions [but] she rejected all these, and adhered literally to her first statement." Once her tests had been passed, Sophia firmly believed in her witnesses and accepted the truth of their testimony.

Sophia's openness required a completely different view of words and their relations to meaning than that I had found in Augustus's logic. Her sources were so diverse that she could not insist on the exact meanings of stories, much less words, in making sense of their statements. She engaged this problem first and most pressingly in the case of the mediums who were the conduit for all of her conversations with spirits. Early on, a medium relayed the message: *"Dear Esther is with me, and we long to clasp you in our arms in this bright world of glory."* Sophia was convinced by the accuracy of the names used that the message was from her father, but she had to confess that " *'clasp you in our arms,' &c.,* was so wholly unlike any language used by my relations when with us, that it puzzled me." She had a similar problem at another session, when her father wrote to her through the medium, but "'beautiful' was *'butiful,'* 'writing' *'riting'* &c." Sophia's efforts to give credence to these utterances led her to see that "the communications were always given in the spelling and phraseology of the person through whose agency they come."

That words did not have fixed and definite meanings meant that, for Sophia, listening was an active process, and understanding was as much a function of a listener's internal state as it was of the words that he or she was trying to decipher; "the Word [of God] itself needs *something* in the recipient to make it effective." She could be quite fierce about those who, instead of constructively listening, were critical of what others said. In her view, their problems lay "in their own inadequate conception."

I found much that was true in Sophia's two-way epistemology. Still, by the three hundred nineteenth page of her book, where she notes "I have already made large demands on my reader's power of belief," I had to admit she was right. Both Sophia and Augustus were convinced of the reality of scenes like that in which "a mahogany dining-table" rose "evenly a few inches from the floor, remaining raised while the friend who accompanied me placed his hand under one castor, and I had mine under that which stood diagonally opposite." I, however, was not persuaded and I did not want to watch Sophia crawl under her dining room table to show that her spiritual understanding could be empirically supported. I wanted to find the Sophia I had so far only glimpsed: the young bride who had been so overwhelmed by her little Alice, the powerful matron who wrote so calmly and sat so peacefully in my only picture.

I realized I was not going to gain access to this Sophia by reading her published works. In the *Memoir* and her autobiography, her construal of the public/private split necessitated that she all but erase herself; in *From Matter to Spirit* it required that she speak from scientific evidence. But I had one other option; I had been told that there was a stash of Sophia's letters in the Lady Byron correspondence in Oxford. Her letters would be private, so I had hopes that there I might find the Sophia I was looking for.

That the corrrespondence existed at all was a somewhat odd idea. I knew Lady Byron only as the controversial estranged wife of the irresistibly sexy, romantic, and rather mad Lord Byron. That she would carry on a correspondence with the resolutely middle-class Sophia seemed unlikely. But William Frend was Lady Byron's tutor before she became Lady Byron, and Augustus tutored her wildly brilliant daughter, Ada Lovelace. As Frend's daughter, Sophia began writing to Lady Byron a decade before she married Augustus, and she continued to do so after their marriage; in the end, the two women's letters would span almost thirty years. So as soon as school was out, I pulled together all of my resources and made a short trip to Oxford.

The archive was at first a disappointment. Lady Byron had kept piles of letters, but not the ones I wanted. There were letters from others in Sophia's family: from her father, William Frend; from her husband, Augustus De Morgan; from her son, William De Morgan. But Lady Byron did not keep Sophia De Morgan's letters; among all these riches I found only two from Sophia. Sophia had kept more than a hundred from her lady friend, though, and at her friend's death the conscientious mother of seven had returned them to Lady Byron's heirs. For lack of anything else to do, I plunged in.

It was a wonderful read. Lady Byron reminded me of Grandmama with her intense involvement in the people around her; her self-conscious, scriptural religiosity; her constant ethical and moral preoccupations. Her world was replete with social causes, financial struggles, and intellectual conundra but also with the everyday. "To my conscience the fulfillment of the slightest relative obligation far exceeds in importance the utility of any scriptural study," Lady Byron explained to Sophia's father as she nursed fifteen-year-old Ada through the measles. Overall Lady Byron's theory of childhood was a kind one: "You could not ask a person more experienced than myself *in error* about the question of whipping little children," she wrote to Sophia when Alice would have been about two. "You might as well attack the cloud in the sky, which whilst you are preparing your assault will vanish away."

Lady Byron did not live in a Newtonian's mathematical universe. Her world was peopled and her space teamed with life. But unlike Sophia, she did not try to meet scientific criteria when she described it.

> Can Science teach that Light and Sound,
> And Motion too, exist around,
>   Yet not by man perceived;
> That Nature fills her realms of air
> With phantoms never dreamed of there,—
>   And this shall be believed?
>
> And canst thou not imagine space
> Peopled with minds whose dwelling place
>   Is not in earthly mould?
> Which undiscerned by mortal eye
> We may not, till to sense we die,
>   With spirit-ken behold.
>
> What this that moment shall renew
> When beings long concealed from view
>   Around shall be discover'd!
> How vain will seem our parting tears
> The oft-waked sighs of lonely years,
>   For those who near us hover'd.

In Lady Byron's world, time did not click by with impersonal precision: rather it flowed and cleansed. "Your feelings of grief form a [veil?] between your mind's eye and her whom you have lost. [Sophia's sister died in the same year that Augustus's did.] But it will be withdrawn, like a mountain mist, and you will then realize the existence of the immortal being.—It has always appeared to me very strange when the bereaved have immediately acquired the spiritual faculty.—To some the conviction that the departed were even witnesses of the survivors' course has come with years—I believed that my Mother lived, but immeasurably remote from me, when she died:—Now I think of her as near, and as perhaps more conscious of my feelings than I am myself.—We must wait for all these changes thro' which our souls have to pass."

These letters, created for me a vivid picture of Augustus and Sophia, not yet married, in two separate rooms of Sophia's father's house. Augustus wrote briskly at his desk calculating probabilities and making reasoned judgments; Sophia gazed out of her window waiting for time and space to reveal themselves and their secrets to her. Neither of them had any question about the reality of the wall that divided their rooms, but I could not see it from my vantage point. From where I stood, invisible in some kind of historian's street, the real included them both.

Within a year of these letters, Augustus and Sophia were married in a civil ceremony. From the beginning it seemed that the men dominated this resolutely radical union: "The idea of the Registrar's Office at first startled the females but by degrees they were reconciled to it," Sophia's father wrote to Lady Byron. However, I saw that it was only together that Augustus and Sophia could understand their world. In some way Augustus knew this: more than twenty five years after the ceremony that had joined them, he would close the "Preface" to his wife's book by saying: "Between us we have, in a certain way, cleared the dish; like that celebrated couple of whom one could eat no fat and the other no lean."

In Oxford, I realized that I had been living for years as if only Augustus's side of the dish mattered. My two years with Ned had forced me to eat from Sophia's side but now I was very poorly equipped to digest it. Neither Sophia nor Augustus was going to be much help in my attempts to understand, though. The wall between the public and the private, the personal and the professional, the wall that had failed me so spectacularly, was essential to both of them. Neither would have been sympathetic to my attempts to incorporate both of their roles into a single life, a single reality.

The issue went beyond sympathy. Augustus and Sophia and the world they had inhabited had defined the very words that I might use to construct a new approach. It was their careful parceling of the world that had left me so frustrated in my attempts to understand and explain. Here again, though, Lady Byron spoke to me. She knew about problems with words.

How are those Theological views to be 'made Known' — ? Not by a *name* or a *phrase* certainly — since to each different hearer that name or phrase will convey a different signification — Witness
"Unitarian — an Atheist
    an Infidel
    a Deist or Philosopher

a Radical or Revolutionist
a rational believer
a 'Christian Hero' (Frend and Tuckerman)"
So that by adopting that name one runs the chance of the most opposite constructions.

What is more, the Lady offered a way to address them:

If then names are unfit instruments for making known our opinions what course is to be pursued? — that of gradually and patiently developing them, as opportunities for such communication may arise. It must be a quiet and private business. There is no medium in my opinion between that and writing a book.

Lady Byron spoke to me in a familiarly firm and well-modulated voice. I listened carefully and as I did my years with Ned became more lived than lost. Even the empty time was not wasted. It all fitted into a purely relative tale, not of logic and probability, but of accident and happenchance.

Afterword (*Nachwort*)

That fall Lady Byron stood by me as I began, gradually and patiently, to develop my lectures and my courses to reflect more fully the whole of the De Morgan platter. It was not easy, and I did not always feel in control, but I did find myself once again able to talk with my students. Then, in January, a year and a half after I had flown away, I returned to Berlin. Officially my trip was to give a seminar at the Max Planck Institute, but really I was going to try once more to close the book, to smooth the sheets and lay the blanket over all.

It was a lightening visit, two weeks snatched between semesters. I arrived on Saturday morning and made my way to my hotel in the *Mitte*, close to the Max Planck Institute. All around the cranes were working their magic. The lowering gray buildings were being removed and transformed into snappy condominiums, department stores, and chic cafés. The domes of the historic churches glittered with new gilt and shiny paint. The streets were still rather empty, but there were more people than before. Berlin was readying itself to become the new capital of Germany; the whole area was holding its breath in expectation of the next great change. Jet-lagged, but unable to sleep, I unpacked my suitcase and contemplated the street outside of my hotel room. Then, carefully, slowly, I moved out into the city.

Berlin was in the midst of its dark winter, but it was unseasonably warm. I left mittens and scarf behind as I moved through *U-Bahn* and bus to the Grunewald. There I found the *See* as peaceful, the *Schloss* as sweet, and the dogs as ubiquitous as ever. I got turned around in the maze of straight paths but easily asked for directions. Then, it was comfortably familiar to walk to lunch with Genie among the matrons in our little café.

The next day, Sunday, I again ventured forth, this time to circle the *Wissenschaftskolleg*. I walked around the Villa Walther, to the grocery store, and down the paths along the *Seen*. The cherubs were still plump, the store still small, the little *Seen* still pristine and wet. The next day, I called Frau Breunig. Then I took the bus to chat with her in the office beside the exotic flowers.

✢ ✢ ✢

On Sunday night, my second evening in Berlin, I called Dr. Walde-meyer. It was good to hear his voice again. The *Kinderabteilung* was going strong, and Drs. Kawalek and Heller were still in the hospital. Petra was gone, though. She had moved to a new job in a clinic that allowed her to work with adults as well as children. Dr. Waldemeyer was clear that the new position was more suited to the variety of her talents, so I was glad. I was sad as well, though. Her absence left a void in my Berlin.

But my Berlin had to be adjusted more drastically as well. The changes that were humming productively around me in the *Mitte* were being less kind to the Otto-Hoffen-Heim. The hospital was going through a massive reorganization and downsizing. Dr. Waldemeyer seemed to feel that his job was secure, as were those of the doctors I asked about, but I could see that the days of Camp Oh-Ha-Ha were numbered. Under the new regime there would be no room for long convalescent stays.

I told Dr. Waldemeyer about Ned's recovery. "Does he come to see us soon?" the man asked, but I had to admit that Ned had no plans to return to Berlin in the near future. "Still, I am glad you called," he said as we hung up.

I was glad too, but as the week went by I realized that I had to go to the Otto-Hoffen-Heim. So very much had happened there. It was a place that I had to see again. I asked around at the Max Planck Institute, and found a volunteer for an afternoon walk. I didn't want to go alone.

Saturday afternoon was unseasonably warm and sunny as Clara and I walked through the Grunewald to the Otto-Hoffen-Heim. We walked to the trailer *Imbis* by the little *Schloss*, and bought *Lumpi*, a sinfully satisfying drink of rum, hot chocolate, and cream. We chatted cheerfully as we sipped and walked through the woods and down the Clayallee.

I had picked the time because I knew that the hospital would be deserted, but still a certain tension descended as we walked past the guard onto the hospital grounds. Nonetheless, Clara was quickly charmed by the pretty little wooded area between the anesthesiology trailer and Station H. I darted into the building, ostensibly to use the bathroom, but really to greet the hot drinks machine. It stood stolidly there, surrounded by its placid plastic chairs.

While I was inside, Clara found a seat in a sunny spot. I returned to find her comfortably leaning back with her feet on a picnic table. At first I was nervous about this breach of propriety; what would the nurses say? But I didn't say anything. Instead I imitated her, and contemplated the hospital over my toes.

"That was my son's window." I pointed.

"Hmmm," she said, noncommittal.

It was the right answer. The window was there, but Ned was not; its time for me was past, its meaning gone. Sitting next to Clara I found myself relaxing into pleasant surroundings and the warm afternoon. We talked for a while about children, hers and mine. Then we took the 110 bus and transferred for one to the *Mitte*.

It was with Frau Sonntag that my nights of solitary German study really paid off. When I called her, she invited me to her house for Sunday afternoon. "I'll show you my apartment and you can meet my husband!" she said, and I could understand her.

So, the day after my trip to the hospital with Clara, I ventured far into the east of Berlin. As I wended my way on unfamiliar *S-Bahnen*, a childhood of Grandmama's tales about Germany and about communism rose up to haunt me. But I made my way without incident and located Frau Sonntag's apartment in the middle of a vast housing complex.

Frau Sonntag and her husband greeted me warmly. They had been on a trip to the United States and were eager to share their impressions. He made a cup of tea for me, and we talked. "They say America is a free country, but everything is forbidden. No smoking! No dogs! No firecrackers! The only thing that is allowed is guns."

"We also cross streets against the lights," I offered.

"But that is dangerous!" Herr Sonntag retorted. We looked at each other for a moment, and laughed. When I had finished my tea, the three of us went for a walk together. We traversed the parking lot behind their building, walked past a field, where perhaps twenty family groups were flying kites, and then up a hill.

"It is a *Trümmerberg*, a rubbish hill," Herr Sonntag explained, when I asked about the unusual phenomenon on the Berlin plain. "They covered over the ruins with dirt and planted grass and trees on it. This is where our children played when they were young."

"It would be fun for Ned to play here, too," Frau Sonntag offered. "If it were a cold winter he could slide down the hill the way my children used to do. If he came again, I would take the day off and show him Berlin! If he came this year, I could take him to our garden."

The woman's face lit up as she described the small garden plot on the outskirts of the city where for years her family had grown vegetables, flowers, and trees. "We will have it for one more year," she explained. "Then the West Germans who owned it before the war will take it back. It is too bad. I do not think that they even care about gardening. But we had it long enough for the children to grow up."

I could not find anything to say, but Frau Sonntag had no intention of being negative. She pointed to the nondescript building in which her tiny apartment was embedded. "You can see our kitchen window from here," she said. "When my children were young, like Ned, we had a big doll. When it was time for dinner, we would put it up in the window. Then the children could see it and they knew it was time to come home." She smiled as she looked towards her kitchen. "The trees have grown so much, even since the children were small," she observed. "They might have trouble seeing the doll now."

I stood on top of a hill created by the rubble of a disastrous war, and stared through winter trees at the uninspired architecture of an East German housing complex. By my side stood a woman who had loved my little boy back to health, even as the order she had always known was falling apart around her. As I stood in a broken world beside this wholly unbroken woman I stopped seeing Ned fallen and me fallen with him. Instead I saw the love with which we had been caught and cared for by a host of strangers.

At some point in the second week one of my colleagues asked whether I would contribute a book on Augustus De Morgan to a series of scientific biographies he was editing. "No," I said simply, somewhat surprising both of us. "I would be willing to write something about Augustus and *Sophia* De Morgan, though."

"Sophia? His wife? There isn't much on his wife, is there? The series is for students. I was thinking more of the university—his teaching, you know."

It was four-thirty in the afternoon and there was no time for me to gradually and patiently develop an adequate response to his objection. But I knew the way was open. There would be time to learn, time to explain, and time to understand. It might not work as part of his series, but I would write a book.

So the next morning I was serene as I boarded the plane. In Providence the doll was in the window, and I was flying home.

Notes

In these notes I have used the following abbreviations to refer to often cited authors:
ADM for Augustus De Morgan
SEDM for Sophia Elizabeth De Morgan
RLE for Robert Leslie Ellis
WRH for William Rowan Hamilton
WW for William Whewell.

I have abbreviated the most often cited texts as follows:
Graves: Robert Perceval Graves, *Life of Sir William Rowan Hamilton.* London: Longmans, Green, & Co., 1889. Volume 3.
Leibniz-Clarke: H. G. Alexander, ed., *The Leibniz-Clarke Correspondence.* Manchester University Press: Manchester, 1956.
Memoir: Sophia Elizabeth De Morgan, *Memoir of Augustus De Morgan.* London: Longmans, Green and Co., 1882.
Whewell Archive: Trinity College Library, Cambridge England. William Whewell Archive.

14   ". . . five or more be invented?" ADM to WRH, Oct. 23, 1852. Graves, 423.
15   ". . . 'quaternion of colours' very soon." WRH to ADM, Oct. 26, 1852. *Ibid.*
16   ". . . make him a popular doctor." *Memoir,* 17.
      ". . . cannot always command." *Ibid.,* 47–48.
      ". . . thirty years after." *Ibid.,* 20.
      ". . . supply the want for themselves." *Ibid.,* 25.
17   ". . . be here to say it." *Ibid.,* 95–96.
      ". . . plays upon words and puns." *Ibid.,* 54.
      ". . . in search of meaning." [ADM], "Review of George Peacock, *A Treatise on Algebra*" *Quarterly Journal of Education* 9(1835):311.
18   ". . . from looking at the past." [ADM], "Theory of Probabilities" *Encyclopaedia Metropolitana,* ed. Rev. Edward Smedley, Rev. Hugh James Rose, Rev. Henry John Rose. (Cambridge: J. J. Deighton, 1845), 2: 393–394.
      ". . . the contrary be specified." *Ibid.,* 396–397.
      ". . . cannot read in the evenings." Quoted in Adrian Desmond and James Moore, *Darwin* (New York: W. W. Norton & Company, 1991), 257.
25   ". . . to ask the Lord's blessing." Hymn 433, *The Hymnal, 1982: According to the Use of the Episcopal Church* (New York: Church Hymnal Corporation, 1985).
32   ". . . Help now mine unbelief." Mark 9: 24.
37   ". . . and immovable." Isaac Newton, *Sir Isaac Newton's Mathematical Principles of Natural Philosophy and His System of the World,* trans. Andrew Motte, Rev. Florian Cajori (Berkeley: University of California Press, 1962), 1:6.
      ". . . hid from our eyes." Hymn 423, *The Hymnal, 1982.*

38   ". . . nearer to their creator." John Herschel, *A Preliminary Discourse on the Study of Natural Philosophy* (New York: Johnson Reprint Corporation, 1966), 16–17.

40   ". . . more probable?" ADM, "Theory of Probabilities," 393–394.

52   ". . . realized by her father." *Memoir*, 189.
". . . write of these events." *Ibid.*, 189–190.

62   ". . . could not be helped." *Ibid.*, 93.

63   ". . . was the best." *Ibid.*, 108.
". . . *an agreeable lull*." ADM to WRH, Sept. 1, 1852. Graves, 410.
". . . promise and beauty." [SEDM], *Threescore Years and Ten: Reminiscences of the Late Sophia Elizabeth De Morgan*, ed. by her daughter, Mary A. De Morgan (London: Richard Bentley and Son, 1895), 186–188.

64   ". . . roused into activity and interest." *Ibid.*, 188–190.
". . . had one herself." A. M. W. Stirling, *William De Morgan and His Wife.* (New York: Henry Holt and Company, 1922), 42.

65   ". . . *to give me a job!*" *Ibid.*, 47.
". . . could not be, you know." *Ibid.*, 44–45.
". . . exercise of all their faculties." *Memoir*, 94.
". . . backward in her learning." Stirling, *William De Morgan,* 48. In his recent biography of William Frend De Morgan, *Rare Spirit* (London: Constable and Company Ltd., 1997), Mark Hamilton attributes this quotation to Sophia's father on page 12, and claims it was written to Lady Byron when Sophia was a child. He does not give a more complete reference, however, so I cannot check his claim. Since, because of its antifeminine ring, the passage sounds to me more like something Augustus De Morgan would write than it does like William Frend, I am leaving the attribution as I originally found it in Stirling's book.

81   ". . . have no quantity." Isaac Newton, *Mathematical Principles,* 1:6–7.

82   ". . . organ to perceive things by." *Leibniz-Clarke,* 11.
". . . you ascribe to him." *Ibid.*, 190

83   ". . . but in vain." *Ibid.*, 191.
". . . imperfection of God" *Ibid.*, 193.
". . . inference would be right." *Ibid.*, 26–27.
". . . order of things among themselves." *Ibid.*, 25–26.

97   ". . . appeal to her mother about it." *Memoir*, 197–198.

118   ". . . conditions of the question?" RLE, "On the Foundations of the Theory of Probabilities" [Read Feb. 14, 1842] *Transactions of the Cambridge Philosophical Society* 8:4.
". . . he was with in life." RLE Diary, March 4, [1836?]. Whewell Archive, Add. Ms. a. 219[6].

119   ". . . before the final separation comes." RLE to James D. Forbes, Sept. 20, 1849. University of St Andrews, James D. Forbes Archive, Ms. 89.
". . . skirts or gaiters etc." RLE to William Walton, [April or May ?], 1850. Whewell Archive, Add. Ms. c. 67[8].
". . . withering cheers me." RLE to [William Walton?], no date. Whewell Archive, Add. Ms. c. 67[57].
". . . died before this hour." RLE letter, Jan 12, 1848. Whewell Archive, Add. Ms. c. 67[9].
". . . ever see you again." RLE to [William Walton?], Nov. 1857. Whewell Archive, Add. Ms. c. 67[30].

120   ". . . if ever anywhere," RLE to [William Walton?], Feb. 22, 1859. Whewell Archive, Add. Ms. c. 67[45].
". . . of life." RLE, "Remarks on the Fundamental Principle of the Theory of Probabilities," [read Nov. 13, 1854] *Transactions of the Cambridge Philosophical Society* 9: 605.

120 ". . . almost perfect moral nature." *Memoir*, 103.
121 ". . . he contemplates." Quoted above, p. 173.
122 ". . . pomp he loves so much." W. H. Wilkins, *Caroline the Illustrious*, (London: Longmans, Green, and Co., 1904), 28.
137 ". . . conscience of the king." *Hamlet*, act 2, sc. 2, lines 603–610.
138 ". . . closely related to fact." William Shakespeare, *Hamlet*, ed. by T. J. B. Spencer (London: Penguin Books, 1980), 265.
". . . *purement*," *Leibniz-Clarke*, 25, n. 3.
141 ". . . for the first time." James Thurber, *The Thirteen Clocks*, (New York: Simon and Schuster, 1950), 31.
". . . by accident and happenchance." *Ibid.*, 32.
". . . was mermaids." *Ibid.*, 43.
165 ". . . 'but it did not hurt.'" Graves, 369–370.
204 ". . . To be a Phoenix . . ." Quoted in Thomas S. Kuhn, *The Copernican Revolution*. (Cambridge, Ma: Harvard University Press, 1959), 194.
234 ". . . what the deuce is that to me?" ADM to WW, Oct. 15, 1863. Whewell Archive, Add. Ms. a. 202[152]
235 ". . . to have their hair brushed . . ." ADM to Sir John Herschel, Herschel Archive of the Royal Society.
". . . which is all one . . ." ADM to Sir John Herschel, Herschel Archive of the Royal Society.
". . . which may assail us." Quoted above p. 118.
236 ". . . hold them by different hooks." ADM to WW, April 30, 1844. Whewell Archive, Add. Ms. a. 202[100].
". . . with mere abstractions." RLE letter. Dec., 1841. Whewell Archive, Add. Ms. a. 222[2].
". . . pinched with cold." RLE letter. [No date.] Whewell Archive, Add. Ms. c 67[82].
"Dec 9, 1853" Whewell Archive, Add. Ms. a. 202[125].
242 ". . . it does not fix my attention." ADM to WRH, April 29, 1854. Graves, 479.
". . . distinguish man from the brute creation." ADM, "Introductory Lecture on the opening of the University of London." University College, De Morgan archive. MS ADD 3:3.
". . . classification by rule." *Memoir*, 98.
"exceedingly humorous" *Ibid.*
243 ". . . connection of thought and language." ADM, *Formal Logic* (1847) (London: The Open Court Company, 1926), 29.
". . . in which they are expressed." *Ibid.*, 31.
". . . if not, introduce it." ADM, "On the Syllogism, No. III, and on Logic in General," [Read Feb. 8, 1858] *Transactions of the Cambridge Philosophical Society* 10: 177.
244 ". . . every linen-draper's shop," *Formal Logic*, 39.
". . . *degrees of knowledge*." *Ibid.*, 197.
". . . it *must* be so." *Ibid.*, 37.
". . . it will not happen." *Ibid.*, 199.
". . . state of imperfect knowledge." *Ibid.*, 200.
245 ". . . to rely upon, trust." *Oxford English Dictionary*, s.v. "believe."
246 ". . . the more evident it seems." ADM to WRH, Oct. 23, 1852. Graves, 423.
". . . anything I see more clearly." ADM to WW, Dec. 9, 1853. Whewell Archive, Add. Ms. a. 202[125].
". . . settled in your own mind." *Ibid.*
". . . philosophy of science altogether." RLE to J. D. Forbes, Sept. 3, 1849. Forbes Archive. University of St. Andrews.
247 ". . . can't get through him," ADM to WW, April 1, 1849. Whewell Archive, Add. Ms. a. 202[113].

247 ". . . sure of finding something." ADM to George Boole, Aug. 8, 1863. G. C. Smith, *The Boole-De Morgan Correspondence: 1842-64.* (Oxford, Clarendon Press, 1982), 114.

". . . speak on subjects like this." *Ibid.*, 102.

". . . I can speak on logic . . ." *Ibid.*, 103.

248 ". . . when I first heard people mention it." *Memoir.* 370.

". . . not voting at all." *Ibid.*

256 ". . . nearly concerned his family." *Ibid.*, 400.

". . . make the presents." WRH to ADM, August 11, 1852. Graves, 401.

". . . never invented those logarithms." ADM to WRH, May 6, 1852. Graves, 357.

257 ". . . she understands them all." WRH to ADM, Dec. 17, 1853. Graves, 469–470.

262 ". . . A. De Morgan" Trinity College Archives, Dublin. MS 1493, 767.

263 ". . . set down again at my desk." Trinity College Archives, Dublin. MS 1493, 772.

". . . *I cannot write of these events.*" Quoted above, p. 74.

". . . sent in his resignation." *Memoir,* 339.

264 ". . . close of the current session was accepted.'" *Ibid.*, 345.

". . . so does my wife." *Ibid.*, 377.

". . . sustained effort." *Ibid.*, 364.

". . . different versions and translations." *Ibid.*, 364.

". . . breathed his last." *Ibid.*, 367–368.

265 ". . . and initials changed." C. D. [SEDM], *From Matter to Spirit,* with a preface by A. B. [ADM] (London: Longman, Green Longman, Roberts, & Green, 1863), 1.

". . . whom she calls [grandfather]." *Ibid.*, 62.

"There is Ellen and M—[Sophia's father] . . ." *Ibid.*, 65.

266 ". . . things *called* spiritual." *Ibid.*, v.

". . . has yet been suggested." *Ibid.*

". . . striven against progress." *Ibid.*, xviii.

". . . what the other had written." *Ibid.*, xlv.

". . . earnest and truth-loving spirit." *Ibid.*, 28.

". . . Byron, Cheops, and Mr. Fauntleroy." *Ibid.*, 27.

267 ". . . to her first statement." *Ibid.*, 185.

". . . it puzzled me." *Ibid.*, 15.

". . . 'writing' 'riting' &c." *Ibid.*, p. 23.

". . . through whose agency they come." *Ibid.*, 16.

". . . to make it effective." *Ibid.*, 357.

". . . own inadequate conception." *Ibid.*, 194.

". . . reader's power of belief." *Ibid.*, 319.

". . . stood diagonally opposite." *Ibid.* 94.

268 ". . . of any scriptural study." Lady Noel Byron to William Frend, June 29, [1829(?)]. Lady Byron papers, Oxford University Library. Box 71, folios 51–52.

". . . will vanish away." Lady Noel Byron to SEDM, March 1840. Lady Byron papers, Oxford University Library. Box 67, folios 104–105.

269 ". . . those who near us hover'd." Lady Noel Byron to SEDM, July 13, [1836(?)]. Lady Byron papers, Oxford University Library. Box 67, folios 79–80.

". . . our souls have to pass." Lady Noel Byron to Sophia De Morgan, June 15, [1836(?)]. Lady Byron papers, Oxford University Library. Box 67, folios 77–78.

270 ". . . they were reconciled to it." William Frend to Lady Noel Byron, Aug.3, 1837. Lady Byron papers, Oxford University Library. Box 71, folios 102–103.

". . . and the other no lean." C. D. [SEDM], *From Matter to Spirit,* xlv.

". . . the most opposite constructions." Lady Noel Byron to SEDM, April 16, 1835. Lady Byron papers, Oxford University Library. Box 67, folios 70–71.

271 ". . . writing a book." *Ibid.*

Acknowledgments

It was in Berlin, sometime in the middle of December 1995, that I first realized that I was living in the midst of a novel. This book began as a series of long letters to my mother, in which I tried to describe and thus explain the story's parameters. Writing them sustained me through the darkest hours of that year's sleepless nights. By the time I left Germany, more than six months later, I was carrying almost two hundred pages of epistolary manuscript.

At that point, I thought I was finished, both with the adventure and with the writing, but I was wrong on both counts. As the final chapters of the book attest, the lived story did not release me completely for almost two years to come. The book held me even longer; I was in its thrall, writing, revising, and writing again, for almost three years after my return to the United States.

The debts I incurred over the course of this saga are so numerous that naming them is simply impossible. Most obviously I am indebted to the Dibner Institute in Cambridge, Massachusetts, and the *Wissenshaftskolleg zu Berlin* in Berlin, Germany, both of which supported me through two very challenging years of my life. I am infinitely grateful that there are still institutions in the world that respect the integrity of individual lives and intellectual exploration to the extent that these did. People in both institutions had expected something very different from me than what I have finally produced. I owe them more than I can say for standing by and allowing me to write a book in my own way.

I am similarly indebted to Brown University. During the past three years, in which I stubbornly persisted in writing the book that was in me, I have learned through experience the meaning and value of tenure in twentieth-century America. I hope that what I have produced justifies, in some small measure, the institutional setup that allowed me to write it.

For the De Morgan materials, I am indebted to the librarians and archivists at the London University; at University College, London; at the Royal Society, London; at Trinity College, Cambridge; at the College Archives in Oxford; and at Trinity College, Dublin. Research projects never end, and just as this book was going to press, the people at the De Morgan Foundation in London located Sophia De Morgan's nursery diary. I am grateful for their vigilance on my behalf.

Behind and within institutions stand people, and here any attempt to enumerate my debts breaks down completely. In my mind's eye I see crowds of them, from janitors to secretaries to administrators, who, often unwittingly, supported me with a smile, a long conversation, a squeezed hand. They were the people who gave me hope when I most needed it.

I then want to thank the doctors and other medical professionals who appear in the book. They are all disguised under false names, but I have no doubt that each will be able to recognize him- or herself. One after another, in inimitable ways, they played their parts in the story, and I am infinitely grateful to all of them.

Then there is the host of friends, neighbors, and colleagues who have steadfastly stood by me, first through the living and then through the writing of this book. Many of those who lived through it appear on its pages under false names; it does not make sense to reveal their identities now, but I thank them nonetheless. Others contributed at later stages, by reading and commenting on seemingly endless drafts. The list is so long that I must apologize in advance for those I left off. I think of Lundy Braun, Teresa Bigelow, Volker Berghan, Gina Feldberg, Menachem Fisch, Mary Jo Foley, Michael Hobart, Evelyn Fox Keller, Martha Manno, Toby and Theo Page, Margo and Lowell Rubin, Mindy Sobota, Jane and Alec Stephens, Molly Sutphin, and Luke Walden. The "biography group"—Jane Lancaster, Adam Nelson, and Eileen Wharburton—generously supported me in my highly unorthodox approach to their genre; Susan Abrams, Upton Brady, Elliot and Marge Kreiger, Joanne Melish, and Ken Miller all offered extensive comments at particularly crucial moments. Then there is my agent, Sally Brady, who saw a book hidden within my initial letters, and kept the faith as I wrote it. Finally, in the past few months Erika Goldman has revealed to me how wonderfully constructive it can be to work with an editor.

Most of all, I thank my families: the far-flung members of the one I was born into and the more present members of the one I live in day to day. To Victoria Campbell and Goodhue Livingston, I owe unwaveringly solid models of parenting; to my siblings—Barbara Nelson, Robert Livingston, and Peter Livingston—I owe the priceless realization that I am never alone in this world. As for the members of my present family, Rick, Brady, and Ned, I thank you for showing me every day how worthwhile life can be.